NESRINE SOUAYEH
MARIEM Noΰira
FATEN DRIDI

Factors predicting the success of intrauterine inseminations

NESRINE SOUAYEH
MARIEM Nouira
FATEN DRIDI

Factors predicting the success of intrauterine inseminations

Imprint

Any brand names and product names mentioned in this book are subject to trademark, brand or patent protection and are trademarks or registered trademarks of their respective holders. The use of brand names, product names, common names, trade names, product descriptions etc. even without a particular marking in this work is in no way to be construed to mean that such names may be regarded as unrestricted in respect of trademark and brand protection legislation and could thus be used by anyone.

Cover image: www.ingimage.com

This book is a translation from the original published under ISBN 978-620-6-72318-9.

Publisher:
Sciencia Scripts
is a trademark of
Dodo Books Indian Ocean Ltd. and OmniScriptum S.R.L publishing group

120 High Road, East Finchley, London, N2 9ED, United Kingdom
Str. Armeneasca 28/1, office 1, Chisinau MD-2012, Republic of Moldova, Europe
Printed at: see last page
ISBN: 978-620-8-25310-3

Contents

1 INTRODUCTION

Since 2009, the World Health Organisation (WHO) has defined infertility as the inability to achieve pregnancy after one year of regular, unprotected intercourse [1]. Infertility is a global health problem affecting between 8% and 12% of couples of childbearing age worldwide [2] . One way for infertile couples to try and overcome their infertility is to use medically assisted reproduction (MAP). Intrauterine insemination (IUI) is a widely used MPA technique for a wide range of reproductive medicine indications, usually offered prior to in vitro fertilisation (IVF) in many indications [3]. ESHRE's 18th report on assisted reproduction showed that in 2014, a total of 120,789 IUI cycles were performed in 39 European countries [4]. In France, IUI accounted for 32% of all assisted reproduction attempts in 2018 [5]. The standard definition of IUI is a treatment for infertility, which involves the placement of prepared sperm into the uterine cavity at the time of ovulation. This can be done in combination with ovarian stimulation or in a natural cycle. The success of an IUI programme is multifactorial [6] and depends on patient age [7], body mass index [8], duration of infertility [9], and cause of infertility [10]. In addition to patient selection, the choice of stimulation protocol [11], the rank of stimulation, the number of mature follicles [10], sperm parameters [12], support of the luteal phase [13], timing of IUI [14] and sperm preparation methods [15] are also prognostic factors taken into account inconsistently by specialists. Overall pregnancy rates after IUI have varied from 5% to 30% [3,14]. The wide variability of indications and the low pregnancy rates compared with IVF have led many doctors and fertility centres around the world to reject IUI and offer IVF as first-line treatment instead [16]. However, IUI is simple, cheaper [17], less invasive, and more patient-friendly than IVF [18], and remains an option when couples are correctly selected. Whatever treatment is used, couples want to know their chances of success. Therefore, it is important to identify and evaluate the factors that influence the pregnancy rate after IUI [19]. In this study, we sought to identify factors predictive of success in intrauterine insemination (IUI) cycles with spousal sperm, in order to define a specific population that would benefit most from IUI. Our work was carried out at the MPA centre of the main military hospital in Tunis. It looked at four years of IAC practice between January 2016 and January 2020. We counted 328 cycles of CAI performed in 196 couples. The aim of this work was to study the influence of various male and female factors on the results of IAC cycles in terms of clinical pregnancies and thus to determine the factors predicting the success of IAC cycles.

2 METHODS

1. Characteristics of the study :

This is a retrospective and descriptive observational study carried out at the main military hospital in Tunis on 196 couples who had at least one attempt at TSI in our centre over a period of 04 years from January 2016 to January 2020, i.e. 328 TSI cycles recorded.

2. Patients :

2.1. Inclusion criteria :

Our study included infertile couples who were undergoing consultation and for whom CAI was indicated as the first option.

For women :

- An age of 40 or less.
- A normal uterine cavity and at least one healthy, patent tube confirmed by hysterosalpingography.
- A woman who has received treatment for a genital infection.

For men :

- A final progressive motile sperm count recovered after the sperm migration and survival test of at least one million.
- Moderate alteration of sperm parameters.
- A popular treatment for male genital tract infections.

2.2. Non-inclusion criteria :

These criteria were :

- Abandoned cycle due to lack of response to ovarian stimulation
- A conversion from ICSI to IAC

2.3. Exclusion criteria :

- Patients with a major alteration in sperm parameters on the day of the attempt and a final progressive motile sperm count of less than 1 million were excluded from our study.
- Patients who have not undergone hysterosalpingography.
- Patients suffering from severe endometriosis.
- Patients aged >40 years.

2.4. Data collection :

Data were collected from the couples' files and from a computerised file of the MPA centre at the Tunis military hospital.

The parameters studied were :

- The patient's age.
- Antecedents (PCOS, tubal obstruction, cervical pathology, etc.).
- Hormonal assessment on D3 of the cycle (FSH, LH, E2, Prolactin) and possibly AMH.
- The regularity of the menstrual cycle.
- Sperm parameters (concentration, mobility, sperm morphology, treated volume, total number of inseminated progressive motile spermatozoa, treated volume, total number of progressive motile spermatozoa before and after preparation).
- Attempt rank.
- The stimulation protocol uses.
- The number of follicles greater than or equal to 18 mm on the day of onset.
- The thickness of the endometrium in millimetres.
- The insemination procedure (easy/difficult).
- The husband's history and habits (smoking, varicocele).
- The type (primary or secondary) and duration of infertility.

The clinical pregnancy rate per cycle was studied as a function of these different parameters.

2.5.Judging criteria :

The success of the IAC attempt was defined by the occurrence of a clinical pregnancy.

2.6.Statistical analysis :

The data collected were systematically transcribed into a database and analysed using SPSS 25.0 statistical software with Pearson's chi-square tests. For the descriptive study, we calculated absolute frequencies and relative frequencies (percentages) for the qualitative variables. Quantitative variables not following a normal distribution were expressed as medians with the first and 3eme quartiles in square brackets, and those following a normal distribution were expressed as mean ± standard deviations. For the analytical study, the analysis was carried out using chi-square tests[2] , and the ANOVA method. The correlation between the different parameters was established using the Pearson method for quantitative variables and the Spearman method for qualitative variables. The significance level was set at p<0.05.

2.7.Bibliographic research :

The bibliographic search was carried out by consulting the digital data available on PubMed, Science Direct, Google Scholar, etc., as well as Tunisian and foreign doctoral theses, using the key words: intrauterine insemination, pregnancy rate and infertility.

2.8.Ethical aspects :

As the study was retrospective, it had no impact on the quality of care. The results obtained will be made available to all scientists interested in this field, for the benefit of patients. The names of the patients not appearing in this work guarantee medical confidentiality, and clear, signed consent has been obtained for all our couples and for each attempt.

2.9.Conflicts of interest :

We declare that we have no conflict of interest.

3. Methods :

3.1.Pre-IAC assessment :

A pre-IUI infertility assessment was carried out for each couple, comprising an interview, a clinical examination and additional tests.

• Careful questioning is carried out to determine the type and duration of infertility, the couple's medical and surgical history, the duration and regularity of menstrual cycles, the presence of dysmenorrhoea, the presence of galactorrhoea, the presence of erectile dysfunction in order to detect sexual dysfunction, the regularity of sexual relations and the absence of contraception, the patient's gestation and parity.

• An investigation including at least the following additional tests:

For the husband :

• A recent spermogram less than 6 months old and a sperm migration and survival test (SMST).

• A sperm culture with a test for mycoplasma and chlamydia.

For women :

• A basal hormonal work-up is carried out on D3 of the cycle, with FSH (follicle-stimulating hormone), LH (luteinizing hormone), E2 (17beta-oestradiol), PRL (prolactin) and possibly an AMH (anti-mullerian hormone) assay.

• An endovaginal pelvic ultrasound to assess the following: uterine and ovarian morphology, antral follicle count, and to check for the absence of cysts, adnexal masses or other findings.

• A hysterosalpingogram carried out in the first half of the cycle (between D7 and D14 of the cycle) and after a negative beta HCG assay.

- A vaginal swab to test for mycoplasma and chlamydia.

For both spouses :

- A systematic infectious disease work-up including serologies for syphilis, hepatitis B and C and the immunodeficiency virus (HIV).

Once the tests have been carried out, the indication for IUI has been established, and all the couples have been informed of the technique and its results, and have signed an informed consent form.

During the couple's final consultation, the doctor explained the IAC cycle, answered any questions the couple might have and issued the prescription needed for the treatment.

3.2.How the CAI cycle works :

3.2.1. Ovarian stimulation :

Two ovarian stimulation protocols with a view to IUI have been used in our department: either clomiphene citrate (CC) alone administered at a dose of 50 to 150 mg/d from 2eme to 6eme days of the menstrual cycle, depending on the patient's hormonal profile. Or CC or letrozole from 2eme to 6eme day of the menstrual cycle, followed by the use of gonadotropins from 7eme to the day before the onset of labour.

The gonadotropins used during the study period were :

J Human menopausal gonadotropins: HMG (Human Menopausal Gonadotropin) Menopur®, Merional®.

J FSH recombinant (FSHr) (follicle stimulating hormone); Gonal F®.

J Highly purified FSH: Fostimon®.

Injections could be daily or scheduled every other day, and had to be given at the same time each day. Doses were usually minimal (between 75 and 150 units/day) and were determined by the patient's characteristics (age, ovarian reserve, BMI, response to previous stimulations and indication for IUI).

3.2.2. Monitoring ovulation :

Three ultrasound monitoring sessions were generally carried out for all patients, the first starting between days 4eme and 7eme of the cycle and then every two to four days depending on response, while adjusting the dose of treatment. This monitoring made it possible to count and measure the diameter of the follicle(s) recruited and to assess the thickness and appearance of the endometrium.

3.2.3. Inducing ovulation :

When one or two follicles had reached a size of 18 mm in diameter, induction was performed by an intramuscular injection of 5000 IU of urinary HCG (human chorionic gonadotropin) or a subcutaneous injection of recombinant HCG (ovitrelin 250 pg).

3.2.4. Act of the IIU :

The partner went to the MAP laboratory to collect sperm by masturbation in an appropriate single-use, wide-mouth receptacle after three to five days of sexual abstinence. The semen was immediately prepared after liquefaction, and a rapid initial evaluation of the sperm was carried out.

sperm parameters was performed in accordance with WHO 2010 criteria. Subsequently, sperm was processed using the 90% and 45% double-layer density gradient centrifugation and migration technique. This consisted of delicately depositing liquefied semen on the density gradient, i.e. 1 ml of each gradient (Sperm-Grad*, 90% fraction and 45% fraction). An initial centrifugation for 20 minutes is carried out at 300-400g. The supernatant was then decanted, retaining part of the 90% layer containing migrated spermatozoa. This fraction was then poured into another conical-bottomed tube containing 3 to 5 ml of sperm nutrient medium (GIVF*, vitrolife), the whole being homogenised, and a second centrifugation-wash was carried out for 10 minutes at 600g. The supernatant was again removed, leaving only the sperm pellet selected in approximately 300 pl or 200 pl of medium (Figure 1).

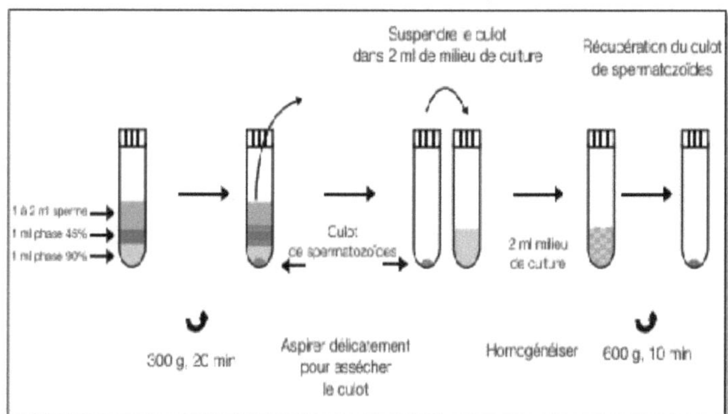

Figure 1: Centrifugation-migration technique on a
90%-45% double-layer density gradient

Insemination itself was carried out 34 to 36 hours after the onset of ovulation. The sperm was injected very slowly, without touching the uterine fundus, in order to avoid reflux and uterine contractions. The patient lay still for 10 minutes.

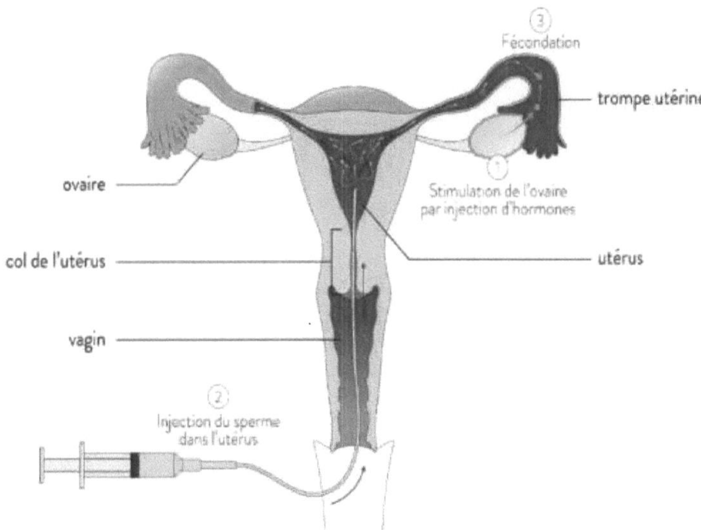

Figure 2: Insemination of prepared sperm in the uterine cavity

3.2.5. Support for the luteal phase :

Supportive treatment of the luteal phase with progestins (Utrogestan® or Estima®) was systematically administered vaginally in all cases at a dose of 600 mg per day.

This treatment was started on the day of insemination and continued for 15 days. It was extended if pregnancy was detected.

3.2.6. Diagnosis of pregnancy :

A quantitative eHCG assay was performed in the absence of menstruation 14 days after insemination. An eHCG level >10 IU/l was considered positive. A clinical pregnancy was defined by an eHCG level > 1000 IU/l and/or evidence of a gestational sac on ultrasound, whereas a biochemical pregnancy was defined by a transient elevation of the eHCG level without resulting in a clinical pregnancy.

3 RESULTS

1. Characteristics of the population studied :

1.1. Female parameters :

1.1.1. A woman's age:

The average age of the women in the CAI cycles was 32.89 ±4.29 years, with extremes ranging from 20 to 40 years. 40.5% of CAIs (133 attempts) were performed in women aged between 30 and 35 years (Figure 3).

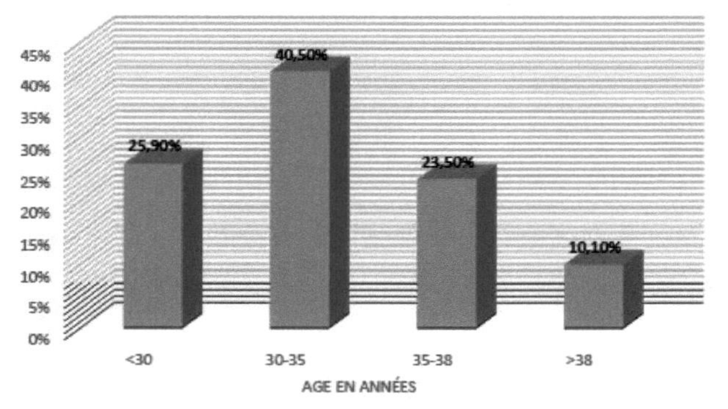

Figure 3: Breakdown of the population by age group in years

1.1.2. Antecedents :

Personal antecedents of medical conditions were present in 22.9% of women. The following table shows the distribution of patients according to their antecedents (Table I).

Table I: Distribution of patients according to their antecedents

ATCD	Number of patients	Percentage (%)
Diabetes	4	1,2
Uterine malformation	2	0,6
Hypothyroidism	3	0,91
Uterine fibroid	7	2,1
Ovarian hyperstimulation	1	0,3
Extra uterine pregnancy	26	7,9
Adenomyosis	2	0,6
Total	45	22,9

1.1.3. Basal FSH assay :

The mean basal FSH value was 7.21±2.99 IU/l with extremes ranging from 1.37 to 21 IU/l. 66 patients had an FSH >9IU/l, i.e. 20.1% (Figure 4).

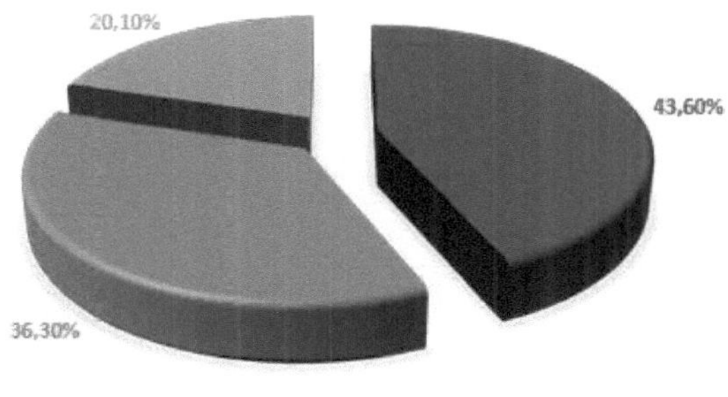

Figure 4: Distribution of the population according to basal FSH level

1.1.4. Basal LH assay :

The mean LH level was 5.20 ± 3.45 IU/l, with extremes ranging from 0.92 to 25.55 IU/l. As measurement of this parameter is not systematic, the LH value was missing in 28% of cases (94 IUI cycles).

1.1.5. Plasma estradiol is measured on D3 :

The mean estradiol level was 50.39 ±21.56 with extremes of 2.5 and 120 pg/ml. Only 7.4% of patients had a high plasma estradiol level >80 pg/ml (Figure 5).

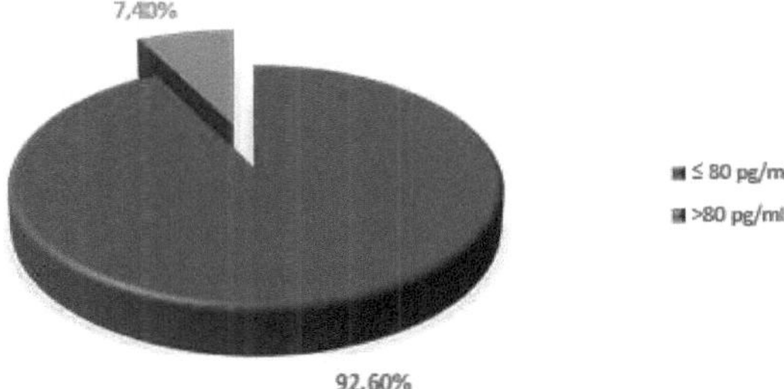

Figure 5: Distribution of the population according to basal estradiol level

1.1.6. AMH assay :

The initial AMH assay as part of fertility testing was not requested systematically, but only in 208 cycles (63% of cycles). The mean AMH value was 3.11 ± 2.77 ng/ml with extremes ranging from 0.33 to 16 ng/ml. AMH levels were between 1 and 4.5 ng/ml in 40% of patients (n=133) (Figure 6).

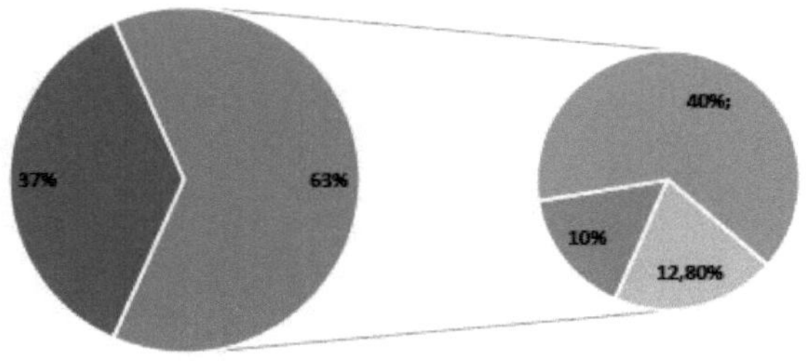

Figure 6 : Distribution of the population according to AMH level

1.1.7. Hyperprolactinemia :

9.8% of our patients (32 IUI cycles) were being treated for hyperprolactinemia.

1.1.8. Regularity of menstrual cycles:

The menstrual cycle was regular in more than 50% of cases (Figure 7).

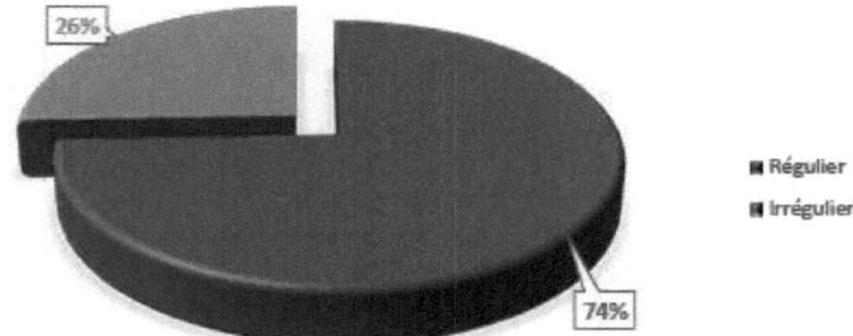

Figure 7: Distribution of the population according to the regularity of menstrual cycles

1.1.9. Hysterosalpingography (HSG) :

Hysterosalpingography was performed systematically in all patients. It was pathological in 14.02% of cases (n=46). 9.7% of patients had unilateral tubal obstruction (Table II).

Table II: Distribution of patients according to HSG results

HSG	Number of IUIs	Percentage (%)
Normal	282	85,9
Unilateral tubal obstruction	32	9,75
Unilateral hydrosalpinx	2	0,6
Poor peritoneal mixing	2	0,6
Isthmic synechia	10	3,04
Total	328	100

1.1.10. Hysteroscopy :

Hysteroscopy was performed in 40 of our patients (12.2%). This examination was performed on clinical, ultrasound or hysterosalpingographic findings. The results were distributed as shown in Table III:

Table III: Distribution of patients according to hysteroscopy results

Hysteroscopy results	Number (IIU)	Percentage (%)
Normal	11	3,3

Synechia cure	17	5,18
Polypectomy	10	3,04
Submucosal fibroma	2	0,6
Total	40	12,2

1.1.11. Laparoscopy :

Laparoscopy was performed for diagnostic and therapeutic purposes. It was therefore used to visualise tubo-peritoneal lesions, to search for associated anomalies, to check tubal permeability and to carry out the necessary therapeutic procedures. Of our patients, 14.93% (n=49) were investigated by crelioscopy. In our centre, crelioscopy was performed in response to clinical or hysterographic signs. The results were as follows (Table IV).

Table IV: Breakdown of the population according to laparoscopy results

Result of laparoscopy	Number of IUIs	Percentage (%)
Normal	24	7,31
Adherences	08	2,43
Endometriosis	02	0,5
Ovarian dystrophy	04	1,21
Ovarian drilling	02	0,5
Tubal plasty	09	2,74
Total	49	14,93

1.2. Male parameters :

1.2.1. Smoking :

67.4% (221) of patients were smokers.

1.2.2. History of clinical varicocele :

33 patients (10%) presented with clinical varicocele.

1.2.3. Sperm culture :

Sperm cultures taken in our patients were positive in 5% of cases, with the following germs isolated: Mycoplasma, Chlamydia, E. Coli.

1.2.4. Initial sperm parameters :

1.2.4.1.   PH

The mean sperm PH was 7.67 ±0.23 (7.2-8.3).

1.2.4.2.   Ejaculate volume:

The average volume of semen ejaculated was 2.91±1.57ml, with extremes ranging from 0.2 to 9ml.

1.2.4.3.   Initial sperm mobility

a. Total mobility

The mean total sperm mobility of the men included in our series was 33.80% ±13. More than 50% of patients had asthenospermia with total mobility <40%, and only 3% had total mobility >60% (Figure 8).

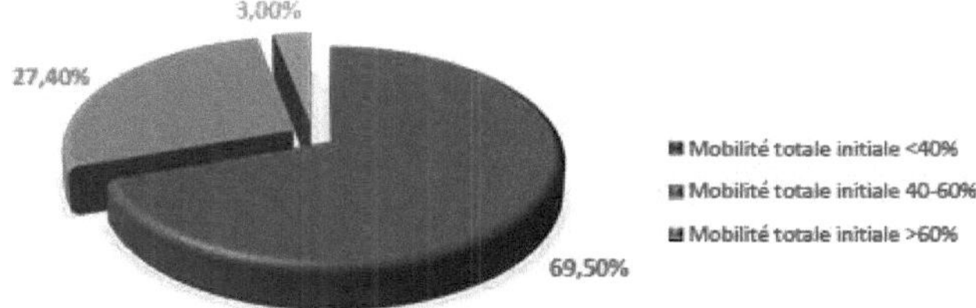

Figure 8: Breakdown of initial total mobility into categories

b. Progressive mobility

The mean progressive mobility was 28.39%±13.6 before preparation (Table V).

Table V: Initial sperm mobility

Initial mobility (%)	Average	Extreme values
Total mobility (a+b+c)	33,8±13	8-75
Progressive mobility (a+b)	28,39±13,6	5-65

69.5% of patients had asthenospermia with progressive mobility <30%. This asthenospermia was severe (<15%) in 10.1% of patients (Figure 9).

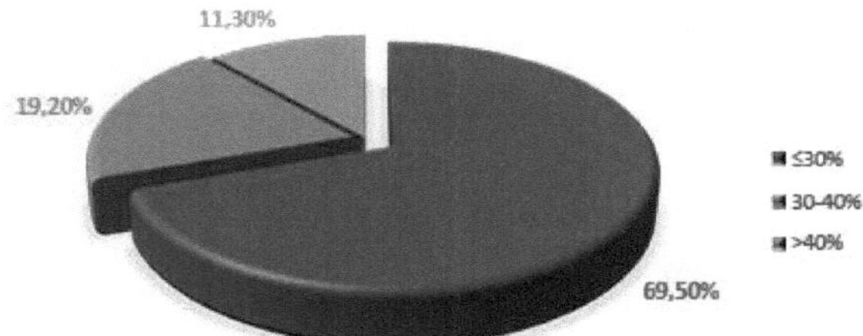

Figure 9: Breakdown of initial progressive mobility into categories

1.2.4.4. Initial sperm concentration :

The mean initial sperm concentration was $53.26 \pm 52.92 \times 10^6$ /ml before preparation (Table VI).

Table VI: Initial sperm concentration

Concentration		
		AverageExtreme values
Initial (x10^6 /ml)		
Before preparation	53,26±52,92	1,3-540

1.2.4.5. Initial total progressive motile sperm count: initial TMSC :

The TMSC was calculated using the following formula:

[Initial concentration (million/ml) x initial progressive mobility x ejaculate volume (ml)] /100

The average value of the TMSC was 35±44 million. We divided the TMSC into four categories as shown in Figure 10:

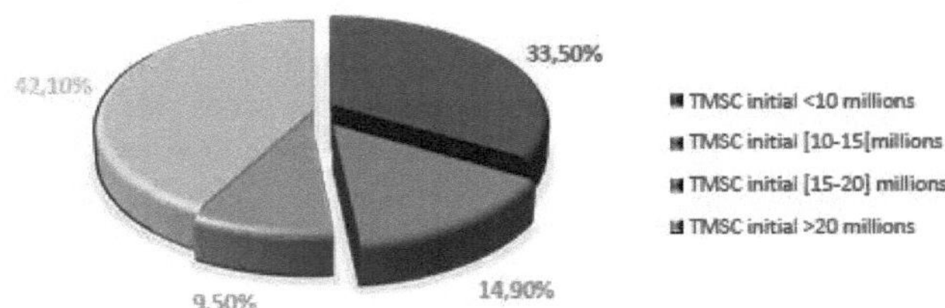

Figure 10: Distribution of IUIs according to initial TMSC rate

1.2.4.6. Sperm morphology

The mean percentage of typical forms (FT) was 14.25±10.46% (2 - 75%).

Sperm morphology was normal (percentage of FT >15% according to the modified David classification) in only 29.60% of cycles (Figure 11).

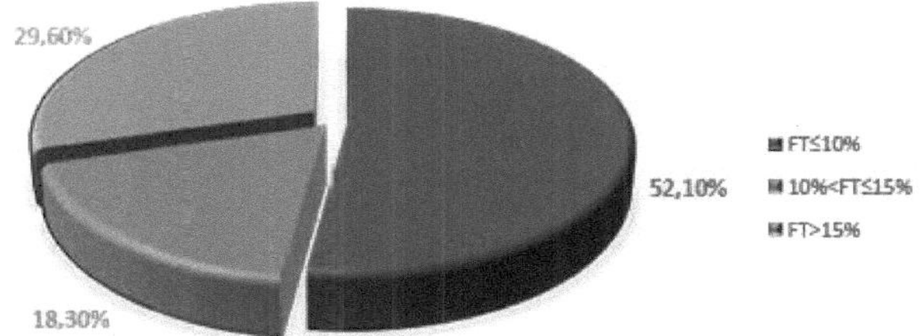

Figure 11: Distribution of CAI cycles according to normal sperm morphology

1.2.5. Sperm parameters after preparation :
1.2.5.1.   Sperm mobility :
a.   Total mobility

Mean total sperm mobility was 75.10%±56 after preparation (Table VII).

b.   Progressive mobility :

Average progressive sperm mobility was 69.91%±15.86 after preparation (Table VII).

Table VII: Total and progressive mobility

Sperm mobility (%)	Average	Extreme values
Total mobility (a+b+c)	75,10±56	10-95
Progressive mobility (a+b)	69,91±15,86	5-97

1.2.5.2.   Sperm concentration :

The mean sperm concentration after preparation was $75\pm56.63\times10^6$ /ml with extremes ranging from 5.5 to 280 million /ml.

1.2.5.3.   The number of final inseminated progressive motile spermatozoa: NSMPI :

The mean value of NSMPI obtained after sperm preparation and selection on the day of IAC was 16.98±14.3 million (1.05-67.2). We divided the CAIs into 4 groups according to the following NSMPI: less than or equal to 5 million, between 5 and 10 million, between 10 and 15 million, between 15 and 20 million and finally greater than 20 million as shown in figure 12.

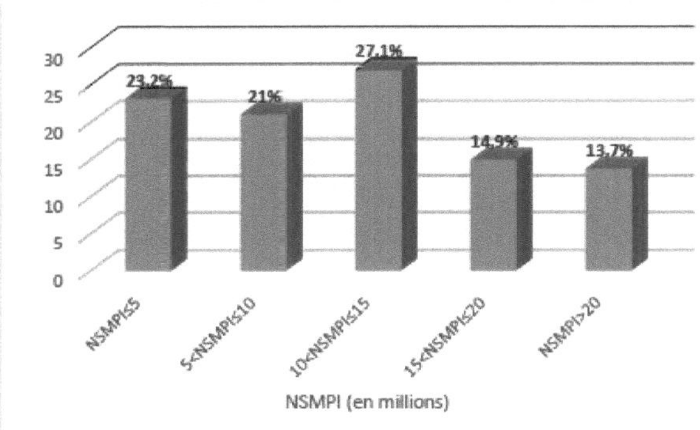

Figure 12: Distribution of NSMPI in our population

1.3. Parameters relating to couples :

1.3.1. Type of infertility :
Infertility was primary in 62.5% of cases (Figure 13).

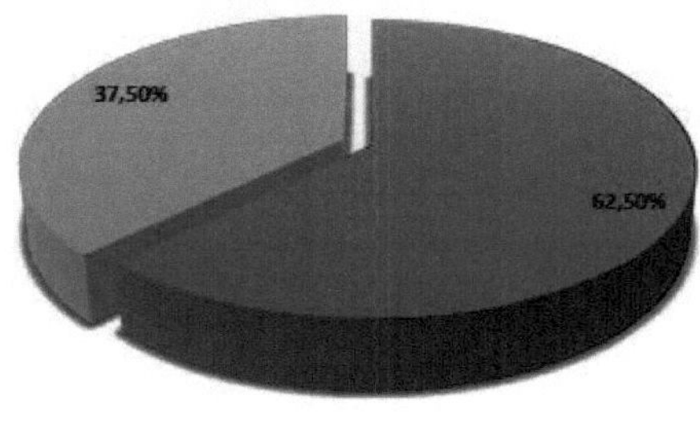

Figure 13 : Distribution of IAC cycles according to type of infertility

1.3.2. Duration of infertility :
The mean duration of infertility in the couples included in this study was 3.3 ± 1.98 years, with extremes ranging from 1 to 11 years. More than half of the couples had been infertile for more than 3 years. The cycles were divided into 3 categories according to the duration of infertility (Figure 14).

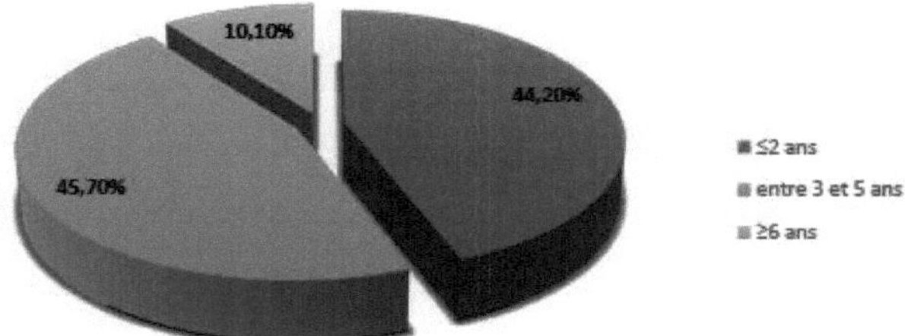

Figure 14: Distribution of IAC cycles by duration of infertility

1.3.3. Indications for TSI :
Almost half of the IACs (44.2%) were carried out for unexplained infertility. In this latter group, the unexplained connotation is relative, because on the one hand the Huhner test (or post-coital test) was not performed, and on the other hand not all patients had benefited from a "closing crelioscopy". In addition, infertility of mixed origin, defined as the association of at least two infertility factors, was present in 9.5% of cases (Figure 15).

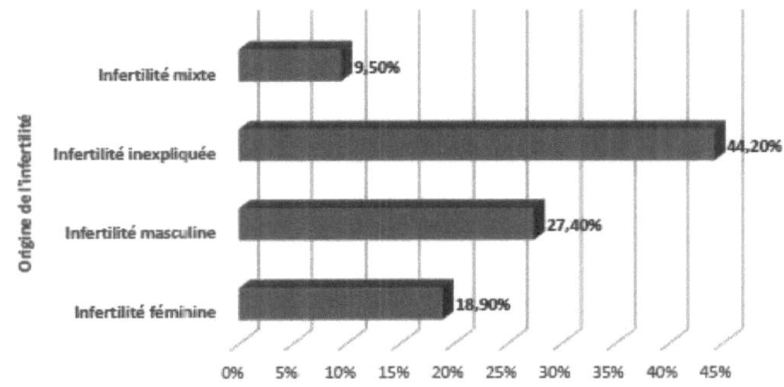

Figure 15 : Distribution of IAC cycles according to origin of infertility

Isolated female indications were present in 18.9% of cases. Polycystic ovary syndrome (PCOS) accounted for more than half of female indications.
Moderate endometriosis and vaginismus were the least frequent indications (Figure 16).

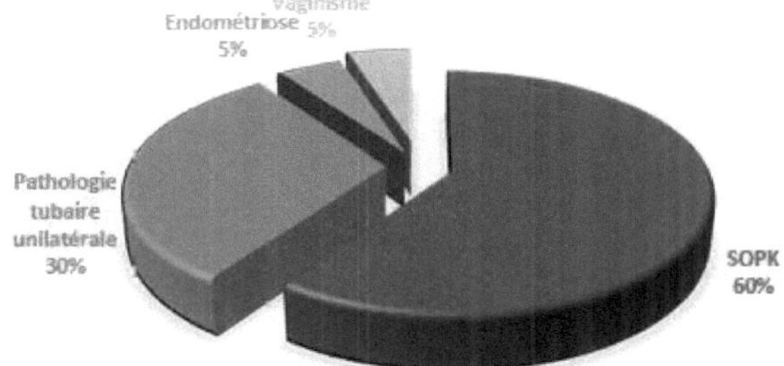

Figure 16: Breakdown of CAI cycles by female indication

1.4. How IAC cycles work :

1.4.1. Number/rank of attempts :

Our study involved 196 couples with a total of 328 IAC cycles.
The majority of our couples (114), i.e. 58.20%, had only had one IUU attempt. Only one couple had had five attempts, and two couples had had six attempts. The average number of attempts per couple was 1.73 (Figure 17).

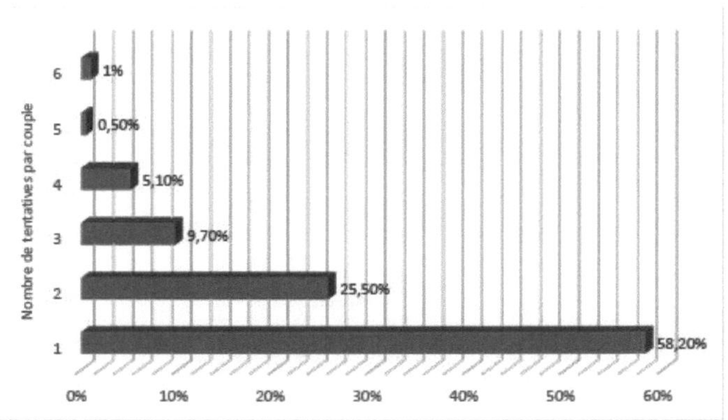

Figure 17 : Breakdown of the number of TSI attempts per couple

1.4.2. Sexual abstinence period :

The mean duration of sexual abstinence before semen collection on the day of the attempted CAI was 3.71 ±1.99 days, with extremes ranging from 0 to 17 days (Figure 18).

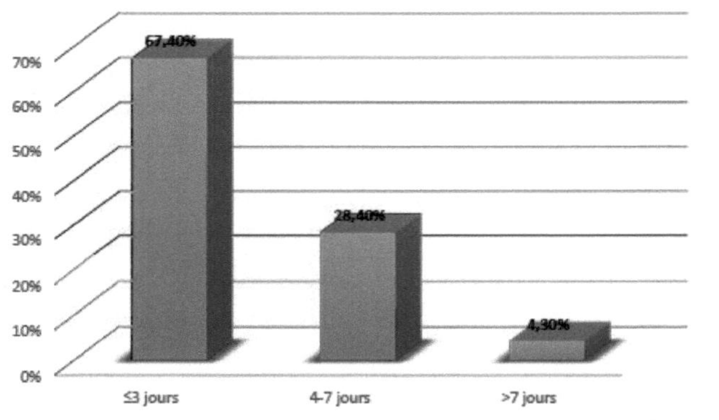

Figure 18: Distribution of IAC cycles according to length of sexual abstinence

1.4.3. Molecules used :

The most commonly used molecules in our study were the association between CC and HMG (43% of IAC cycles) followed by the association between CC and FSH (33.2%) (Figure 19). IUI was spontaneous in only one woman with a history of attempted IUI not performed in our department, complicated by ovarian hyperstimulation syndrome requiring hospitalisation.

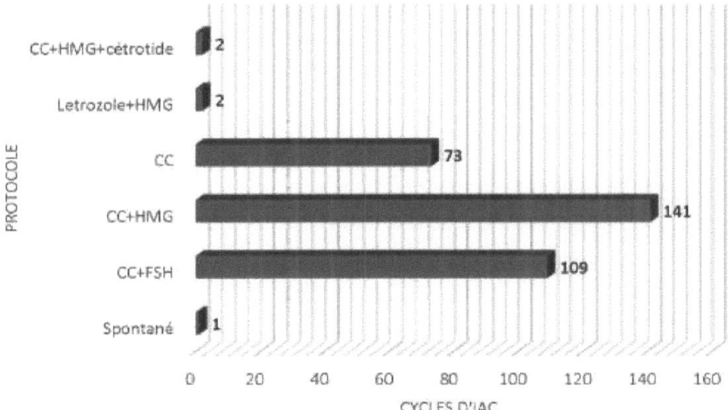

Figure 19: Breakdown of cycles according to protocols used

Over 70% of women with PCOS had benefited from ovarian stimulation using a combination of CC and HMG or FSH (Table VIII).

Table VIII: Compounds used for ovarian stimulation according to the cause of infertility

Origin of infertility	Protocol					
	Spontaneous	CC+Gonadotrophins (FSH or HMG)	CC	Letrozole+HMG	CC+HMG + Cetrotide	Total
Male infertility	0	65 (72,2%)	24 (26,7%)	0	1 (1,1%)	90 (100%)
Unexplained infertility	1	113 (77,9%)	31 (21,4%)	0	0	145 (100%)
Mixed infertility	0	22 (71%)	8 (25,8%)	1 (3,2%)	0	31 (100%)
PCOS	0	28 (75,7%)	8 (21,6%)	0	1 (2,7%)	37 (100%)
Tubal pathology	0	17 (89,5%)	1 (5,3%)	1 (5,3%)	0	19 (100%)
Endometriosis	0	3 (100%)	0	0	0	3 (100%)
Vaginism	0	2 (66,7%)	1 (33,3%)	0	0	3 (100%)
Total	1	250	73	2	2	328

1.4.4. Gonadotropin dose :

The mean dose of gonadotropins used was 359.34±174.82 for HMG and 333.1±174.05 for FSH. The maximum dose was 1500 IU.

1.4.5. Number of mature follicles greater than 18 mm on day of onset:

The mean number of mature follicles obtained on the day of initiation in our study population was 1.96, with extremes of 1 to 4 follicles. Ovarian stimulation was monofollicular in 115 cycles, bi-follicular in 130 cycles and multi-follicular (>2 follicles) in 83 IAC cycles (Figure 20).

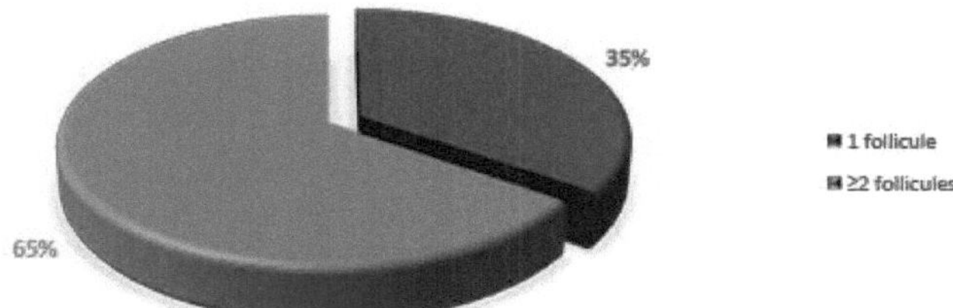

Figure 20: Distribution of CAI cycles according to the number of follicles >18mm

1.4.6. Thickness of the endometrium :

The mean endometrial thickness on the day of induction was 8.88 ±1.76 mm, with extremes of 6 to 15 mm (Figure 21).

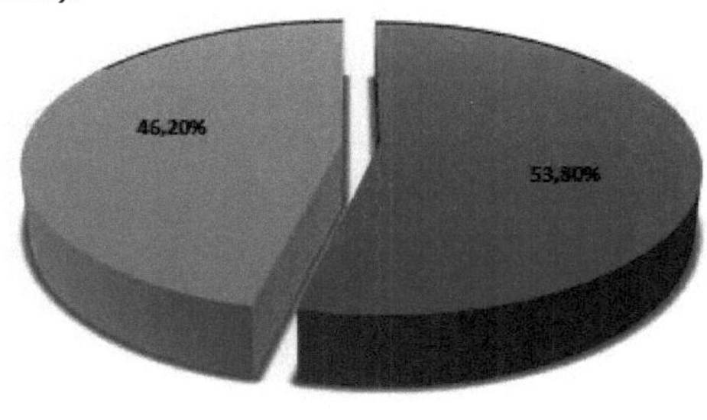

Figure 21: Distribution of CAIs according to endometrial thickness

1.4.7. Quality of the insemination act :

Insemination of spermatozoa prepared inside the uterus was difficult in only 11% of patients (n=36), or a rigid catheter was used (Figure 22).

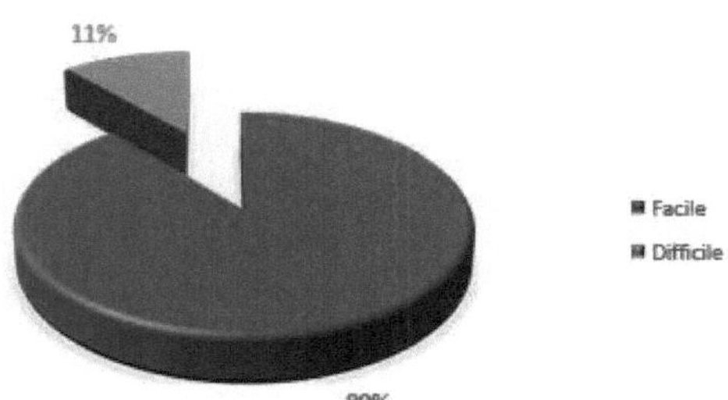

Figure 22 : Distribution of CAI cycles according to the quality of the insemination procedure

1.4.8. Time between semen preparation and insemination :

The average time between sperm preparation and insemination was 30 minutes, with extremes ranging from 10 minutes to 1 hour.

2. Results in terms of pregnancy rate per CAI cycle:

2.1. Overall results :

Of the 328 cycles carried out in 196 couples, 52 pregnancies were obtained, i.e. 15.24% per cycle and 25% per couple. These 52 pregnancies were distributed as follows:

- 50 clinical pregnancies (including one extra-uterine pregnancy).
- 02 biochemical pregnancies.

Of these 50 clinical pregnancies, two were gemellar and one was triple-arrested. The multiple pregnancy rate was therefore 0.9% (Figure 23).

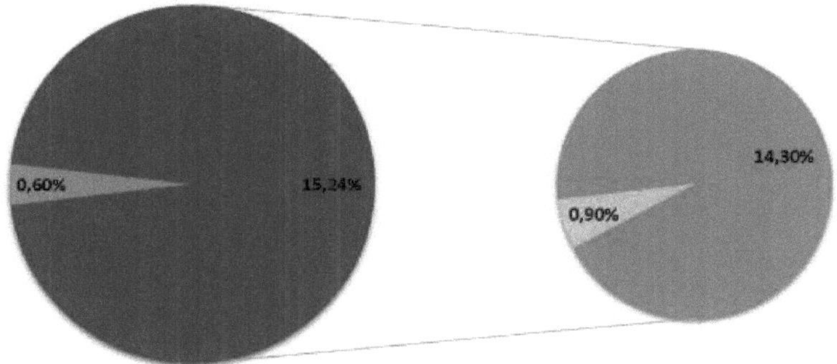

Figure 23: Breakdown of pregnancies obtained in our study

2.2. Resuitats based on female parameters :

2.2.1. Age of the woman

The highest pregnancy rate was found among women aged 30-35, at 16.5%. The difference between the different age groups was not statistically significant.
significant (p= 0.766) (Figure 24).

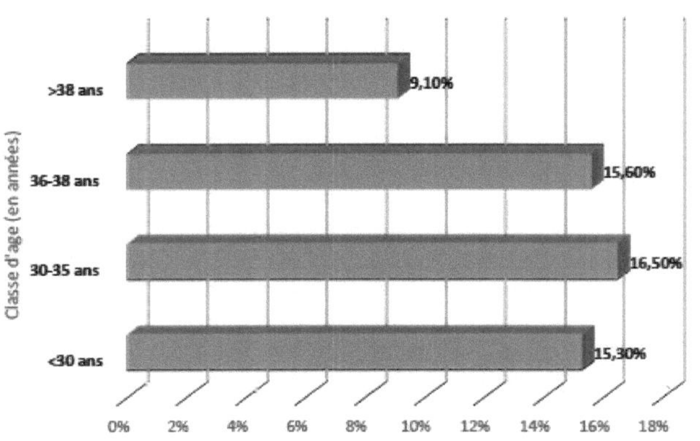

Figure 24: Pregnancy rate as a function of female age

2.2.2.

2.2.3. Determination of basal FSH and LH :

The initial FSH level had a significant influence on the outcome of TSI (**p=0.016**). The results are shown in the figure below (Figure 25):

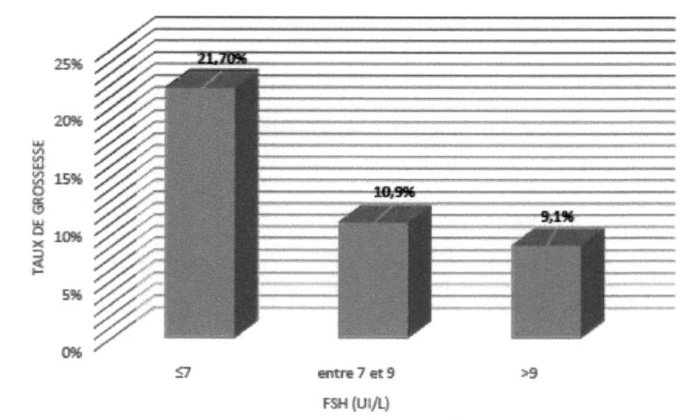

Figure 25: Pregnancy rate as a function of basal FSH

No difference was noted in the pregnancy rates observed according to the basal LH value (p=0.936) (Table IX).

Table IX: Average LH levels according to pregnancy

LH	Pregnancy	No pregnancy	p-value
Average value	5,97±3,56	5,93±3,0	NS p=0,936

2.2.4. AMH :

AMH levels were missing in 120 cycles (i.e. 36% of IAC cycles performed during the study period). The highest pregnancy rate was obtained with an AMH between 1 and 4.5 ng/ml, i.e. 27.1% versus 12.1% and 16.7% with an AMH <1ng/ml and >4.5 ng/ml respectively, but this difference was not significant (p=0.109) (Figure 26).

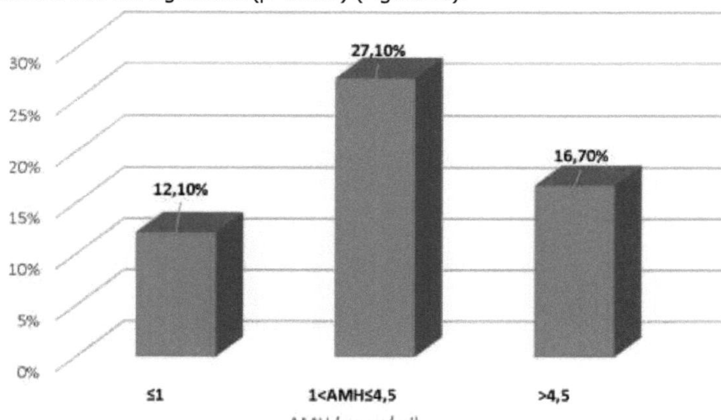

Figure 26: Pregnancy rate as a function of AMH

In fact, AMH had a statically significant impact on the pregnancy rate in women with PCOS. The latter fell from 72.7% when the AMH level was between 1 and 4.5 ng/ml to 26.3% when the AMH level exceeded 4.5 ng/ml (**p=0.032**) (Figure 27).

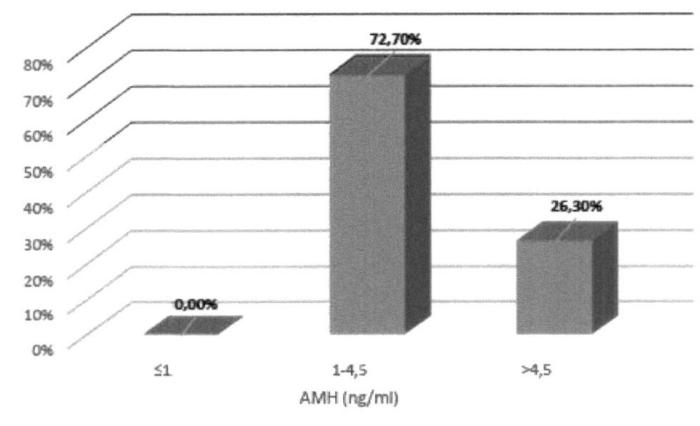

Figure 27: Pregnancy rates in women with PCOS according to AMH

2.2.5. Estradiol levels :

The initial estradiol level did not have a significant influence on the outcome of the IAC (p=0.511). In the 50 pregnancies obtained, estradiol was <80 pg/ml in 93.9% of cases.

2.2.6. Regularity of the menstrual cycle :

The regularity of the menstrual cycle did not appear to influence the outcome of CAI cycles: the pregnancy rate was 13.9% when the cycle was regular compared with 17.9% when it was irregular (p=0.384).

2.3.Results based on couple parameters :

2.3.1. Duration of infertility :

In our study, the duration of infertility had a significant impact on the pregnancy rate (p=0.04). To better study the effect of this parameter on the chances of pregnancy, we divided the study sample into 3 groups according to the duration of infertility: less than or equal to 2 years, 3 to 5 years and more than 5 years of infertility for the couple. There was a significant decrease in the pregnancy rate per cycle as the duration of infertility increased, from 19.3% when the duration of infertility was < 2 years to 14.7% when it was between 3 and 5 years, and no pregnancy when it was over 6 years (**p=0.02**) (Figure 28).

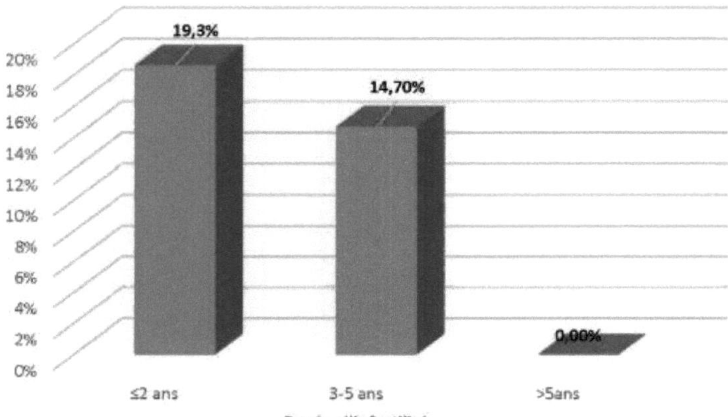

Figure 28: Pregnancy rate per cycle as a function of duration of infertility

2.3.2. Type of infertility :

The difference in terms of pregnancy between primary and secondary infertility was not significant (p= 0.475). Figure 29 summarises the results obtained.

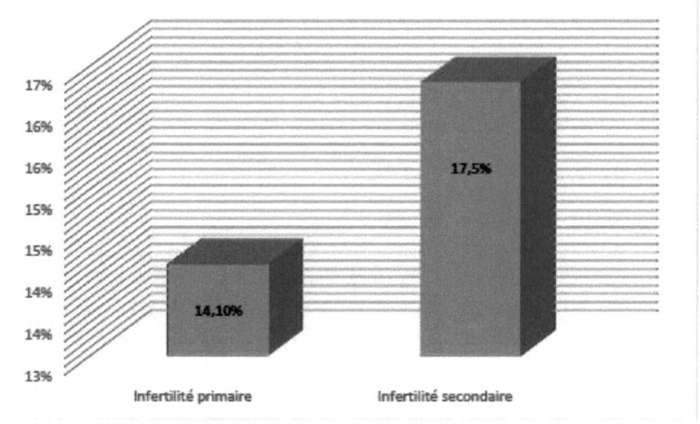

Figure 29: Pregnancy rates by type of infertility

2.3.3. Origin of infertility :
2.3.4.

The best results in terms of clinical pregnancies per cycle were obtained in cases of dysovulatory infertility; PCOS (35.1%) followed by unexplained infertility (14.5%). No pregnancies were obtained in cases of endometriosis or vaginismus. The difference between the different groups was statistically significant (**p=0.024**) (Table X).

Table X: Breakdown of clinical pregnancy rates by cause of infertility

Origin of infertility	Number of TSIs	Pregnancy	p-value
Inexplicable infertility	145	21 (14,5%)	
Male infertility	90	11 (12,2%)	
PCOS	37	13 (35,1%)	

Unilateral tubal pathology	19	2 (10,5%)	**0,024**
Endometriosis	3	0	
Vaginism	3	0	
Mixed infertility	31	3 (9,7%)	

2.4.Results based on male parameters:

2.4.1. History of clinical varicocele :

Clinical varicocele did not have a significant impact on IUI results (p=0.320) (Table XI).

Table XI: Pregnancy rates according to varicocele disease

Varicocele	Pregnancy	No pregnancy	Total	P
Yes	3 (9,1%)	30(90,9%)	33(100%)	0,320
No	47(15,9%)	248(84%)	295(100%)	

2.4.2. Tobacco :

There was no significant difference between male smokers and non-smokers in terms of clinical pregnancy rates (14.5% and 15.8% respectively, p=0.637) (Figure 30).

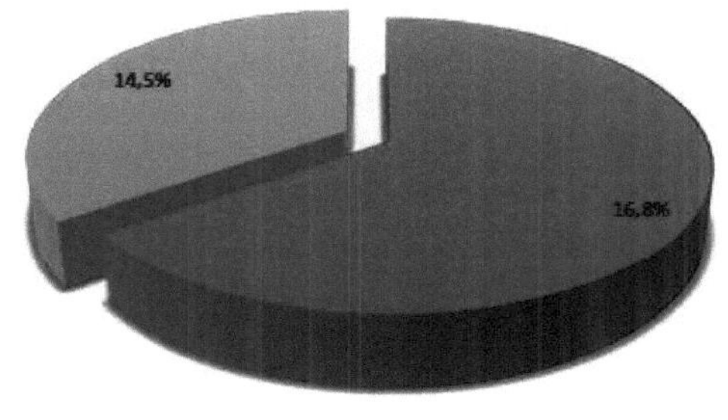

Figure 30: Pregnancy rates according to male smoking habits

2.4.3. Sperm culture :

Of the 16 sperm culture-positive couples treated, four (25%) achieved pregnancy. The sperm culture result did not have a significant impact on IUI results (p=0.27) (Table XII).

Table XII: Pregnancy rate per cycle according to sperm culture result

Sperm culture	Pregnancy	No pregnancy	Total	p-value
Positive	4 (25%)	12 (75%)	16 (100%)	0,27
Negative	46 (14,7%)	276 (85,4%)	312 (100%)	

2.4.4. Initial and post-preparation sperm parameters

2.4.4.1.   Sexual abstinence period :

The highest pregnancy rate was obtained after 4 to 7 days of sexual abstinence. This parameter had no significant influence on the pregnancy rate (p=0.478) (Figure 31).

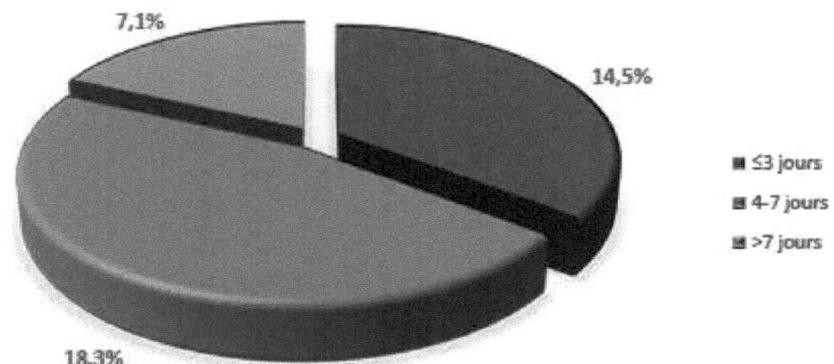

Figure 31: Pregnancy rate according to length of sexual abstinence

2.4.4.2.   PH :

The mean PH was 7.65±0.24 in the case of pregnancy versus 7.68±0.23 in the absence of pregnancy (p=0.579).

2.4.4.3.   Ejaculate volume :

Ejaculate volume had no influence on IUI results. The mean value was 2.6±1.2 ml in the pregnancy group versus 2.7 ±1.6 in the non-pregnancy group (p=0.134).

2.4.4.4.   Sperm mobility :

The comparison of means test showed no difference between total sperm mobility after preparation in women who had become pregnant and those who had not (p=0.939). On the other hand, initial total sperm mobility had a significant and positive impact on pregnancy rates **(p=0.001)**. Similarly, progressive mobility before preparation had an impact on IUI results **(p=0.004)** and there was no significant difference between the mean values of progressive mobility after preparation in the 2 pregnancy and non-pregnancy groups (Table XIII).

Table XIII: Pregnancy rate and sperm mobility

Mobility		Mean +/- standard deviation		p-value
		No pregnancy	Pregnancy	
Total mobility	Initial	32,89±12,9	38,85±17	**0,001**
	After preparation	75±15	75±18	0,939
Progressive mobility	Initial	27,40±12,5	33,86±17,62	**0,004**
	After preparation	72,27±10,1	73,68±10,4	0,996

We divided the initial total mobility into 3 groups: <40%, between 40 and 60% and >60%. There was a statistically significant difference between these groups, with the rate of clinical pregnancy increasing from 11.8% when the initial mobility was <40% to 20% and 50% when the initial total mobility was between 40 and 60%, and >60% respectively **(p=0.002)**. Study of the progressive mobility subgroups showed that there was a statistically significant difference between them, with the pregnancy rate increasing from 11.5% to 35.1% when the initial progressive mobility was <30% and >40% respectively **(p=0.001)**, as shown in the following table XIV:

Table XIV: Pregnancy rates according to initial progressive and total mobility

Mobility initial	Categories	Number of IUIs	Pregnancy	p-value
	<40%	228	27 (11,8%)	

24

Total a+b+C	40-60%	90	18 (20%)	0,002
	>50%	10	5 (50%)	
Progressive - a+b	<30%	226	26 (11,5%)	
	30-40%	65	11 (17%)	0,001
	>40%	37	13 (35,1%	

2.4.4.5. Pregnancy rate as a function of sperm concentration :

In our study, there was no difference in pregnancy rate between the initial sperm concentration and the sperm concentration after preparation on the day of insemination as shown in Table XV.

Table XV: Pregnancy rate and sperm concentration

Average concentration ($\times 10^6$ /ml)	No pregnancy	Pregnancy	p-value
Before preparation	45,7±59,11	51,64±54,83	0,518
After preparation	73±56	86,2±56,8	0,134

2.4.4.6. Initial TMSC :

The highest pregnancy rate was obtained with more than 20 million TMSC, i.e. 27 pregnancies, whereas only 5 pregnancies were obtained when the TMSC was between 10 and 15 million. However, this difference was not significant (p=0.304), as shown in Figure 32 below:

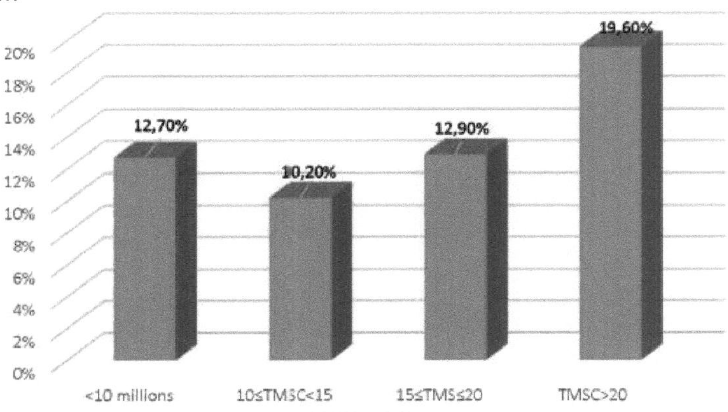

Figure 32: Pregnancy rate and initial MSCR

2.4.4.7. Sperm morphology :

We noted a significant increase in the pregnancy rate when the percentage of typical sperm forms exceeded 15% using the modified David classification, and the pregnancy rate rose from 8.2% to 20% and then 24.7% when the mean percentage of FTs was <10%, between 10 and 15% and >15% respectively (**p=0.001**) (Figure 33).

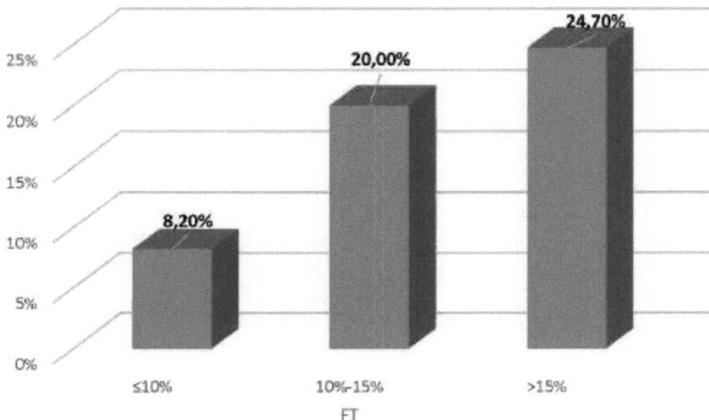

Figure 33: Pregnancy rate and sperm morphology

2.4.4.8.   NSMPI :

An NSMPI of >5 million was associated with a significant increase in the pregnancy rate, i.e. 17.9% compared with 5.3% if the NSMPI was <5 million (**p=0.007**) (Figure 34).

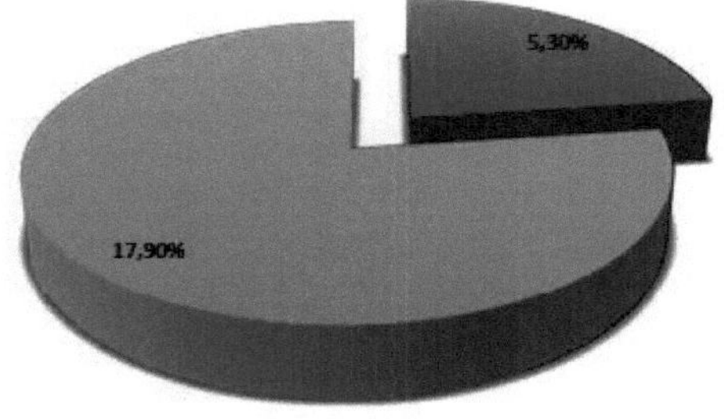

Figure 34: Pregnancy rate per cycle as a function of NSMPI To refine our results, we divided the NSMPI into five intervals. The pregnancy rate per cycle was 26.5% when NSMPI was between 15.1 and 20 million and only 5.3% when NSMPI was <5 million. The difference between the NSMPI groups was also statically significant (**p=0.001**). On the contrary, there was no difference between the NSMPI groups between 15.1 and 20 million and NSMPI >20 million, i.e. a pregnancy rate of 26.5% versus 26.7% respectively (p=0.912) (Figure 35).
30%

26

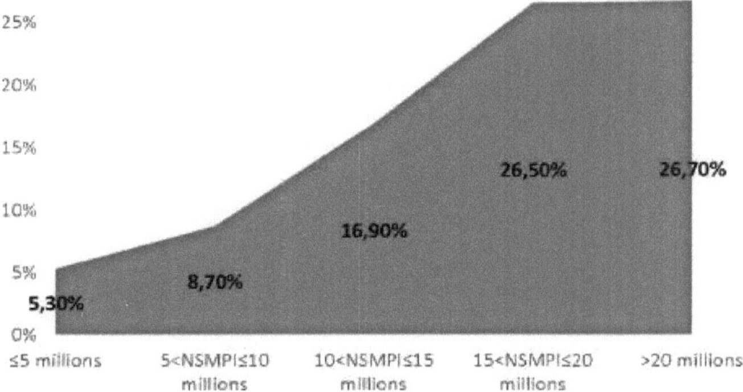

Figure 35: Pregnancy rate and NSMPI

2.5. Results as a function of attempt rank :

At the end of the second attempt, 20 clinical pregnancies were obtained, i.e. 40.8% of clinical pregnancies. No pregnancies were obtained after the 5th attempt. In our series, the number of attempts correlated significantly and negatively with the pregnancy rate after insemination beyond the second attempt **(p =0.000)**, as shown in Figure 36.

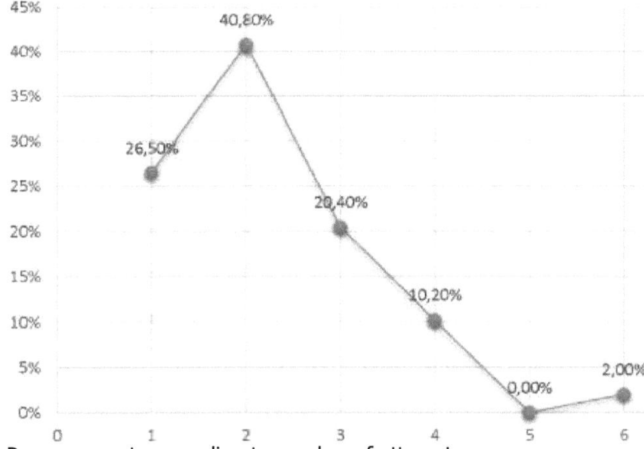

Figure 36: Pregnancy rate according to number of attempts

2.6. Pregnancy rates according to the molecules used :

The highest pregnancy rate was obtained after ovarian stimulation by CC+FSH (19.3%), but the difference was not significant compared with the other molecules used (p=0.469). The use of Letrozole resulted in 50% pregnancy, but this compound was only used in 2 cases, i.e. 0.6% of the cycles studied. The results are presented in Table XVI.

Table XVI: Pregnancy rates according to molecules used

Protocol	Number of IUIs	Pregnancy (%)	p-value
Spontaneous	1	0	
CC+FSH	109	19,3 (21)	
CC+HMG	142	12,7 (18)	0,469
CC	74	13,6 (10)	

2.7. Pregnancy rates as a function of gonadotropin doses :

In our study, there was no difference in pregnancy rates for FSH and HMG doses (Table XVII).

Table XVII: Pregnancy rates and gonadotropin doses

Average dose values for Gonadotropins	Pregnancy	No pregnancy	p-value
FSH	316,88±95,	456336,15±184,150	0 ,522
HMG	359,21±95,	456349,01±184,076	0,813

2.8. Results according to the number of mature follicles >18mm obtained :

The best clinical pregnancy rate per observed cycle was obtained with >2 follicles >18mm, i.e. 18.77% compared with 8.6% after monofollicular stimulation (**p=0.015**) (Figure 37).

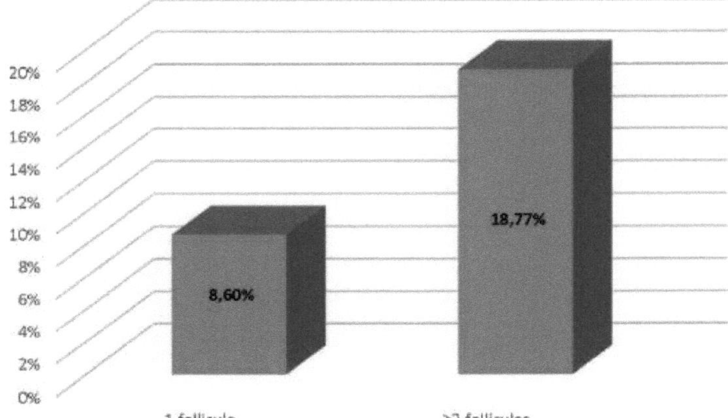

Figure 37: Pregnancy rate as a function of the number of mature follicles

2.9. Results as a function of endometrial thickness on the day of induction:

We divided our population into two groups according to whether the endometrial thickness was greater or less than 9 mm on the day of onset. We found a significant difference in clinical pregnancy rate between the two groups (**p=0.001**) as shown in figure 38.

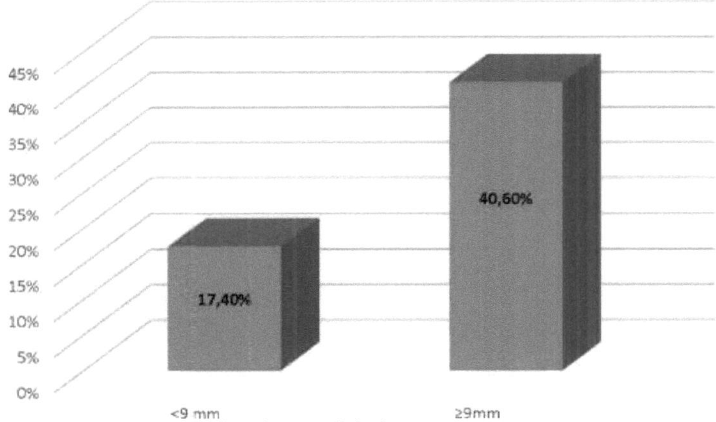

Figure 38: Pregnancy rate and endometrial thickness

2.10. Results according to the quality of the insemination procedure :

Of the 50 pregnancies, only 3 were obtained after difficult insemination. It should be noted that inseminations were difficult in 36 IUI cycles, i.e. 11% of cycles. The difference was not significant (p=0.293) (Figure 39).

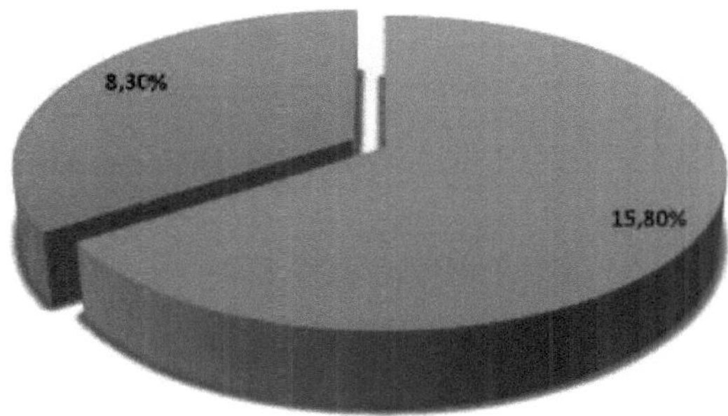

Figure 39: Pregnancy rate according to the quality of the insemination procedure

2.11. Post-insemination complications :

We did not observe any hyperstimulation syndrome in our patients.

6% of the pregnancies obtained were multiple, with two gemellar pregnancies and one multiple pregnancy.

3. Correlative study of clinical and biological factors influencing the success of IUI cycles:

According to our study, the highest pregnancy rates were obtained after 2 years of infertility in the first 2 insemination cycles, in women with an FSH level < 7UI/L suffering from PCOS, with 2 mature follicles and an endometrial thickness >9 mm on the day of onset and adequate sperm parameters, i.e. initial and/or total progressive mobility >40%, percentage of typical forms >15% and NSMPI >5 million.

We found that female age, AMH level, type of infertility, sperm concentration and sperm mobility after preparation had no influence on our results in terms of clinical pregnancy rate

(Table XVIII).

Table XVIII: Correlation between various factors and pregnancy rate

Parameter	Number of cycles	Number of pregnancies	Pregnancy rate (%)	P value
Age of women <30	85	13	15,3	0,755
30-35 years old	133	22	16,5	0,808
Age 36-38	77	12	15,6	0,858
>38 years	33	3	9,1	0,381
FSH (IU/l) <7	143	31	21,7	**0,016**
]7-9]	119	13	10,9	**0,012**
>9	66	6	9,1	**0,027**
AMH (ng/ml) <1	33	4	12,1	0,109
]1-4,5]	133	36	27,1	0,73
>4,5	42	7	16,7	0,58
Duration of infertility (years)				**0,02**
<2	145	28	19,3	0,04
[3-5]	150	22	14,7	**0,006**
>6	33	0	0	
Type of infertility Primary	205	29	14,1	0,475
Secondary	123	21	17,1	
Origin of PCOS infertility	37	13	35,1	**0,024**
Inexplicable infertility	145	21	14,5	**0,02**
Male infertility	90	11	12,2	**0,03**
Mixed infertility	31	3	9,7	**0,54**
Tubal pathology	19	2	10,5	**0,05**
Endomdtriosis	3	0	0	0,492
Vaginism	3	0	0	0,492
Smoking in men				
Yes	221	32	14,5	0,637
No	107	18	16,8	
Initial total mobility (%)				**0,002**
<40	228	27	11,8	
40-60	90	18	20	**0,02**
>60	10	5	50	**0,000**
Initial progressive mobility (%)				**0,001**
<30	226	26	11,5	
30-40	65	11	17	0,2
>40	37	13	35,1	**0,000**
Initial TMSC (millions)	110			0,304
<10		14	12,7	
10-15		5	10,2	0,653
15-20		4	12,9	0,972
>20	138	27	19,6	0,151
Morphology (%)				**0,001**
<10	171	14	8,2	
]10-15]	60	12	20	**0,013**
>15	97	24	24,7	**0,000**
NSMPI (million)				**0,001**
<5	76	4	5,3	
5,1-10	69	6	8,7	0,419
10,1-15	89	15	16,9	**0,02**
15,1-20	49	13	26,5	**0,001**
>20	45	12	26,7	**0,001**
Sexual abstinence period				0,478
<3 days	221	32	14,5	
4-7 days	93	17	18,3	0,399

>7 days	14	1		7,1	0,446
Number of attempts					**0,000**
1	114	13	11,4		
2	50	20	40		**0,000**
3	19	11	57,9		**0,000**
4	10	5	50		**0,001**
5	1	0	0		0,723
6	2	1	50		0,009
Protocol					0,469
CC+FSH	109	21	19,3		
CC+HMG	142	18		12,7	0,161
CC	74	10	13,6		0,330
Letrozol+HMG	2	1	50		0,284
Spontand	1	0	0		0,495
Number of mature follicles					
1	115	10	8,6%		
>2					0,015
	213	40		18,77%	
Endometre thickness (mm)					
<9	115	20	17,4		0,001
	69	28	40,6		

4 DISCUSSION

Intrauterine insemination (IUI) is often the first step in infertility treatment for couples suffering from unexplained infertility, impaired sexual function and mild to moderate male hypofertility. Overall success rates per IUI cycle are rather low compared with other techniques such as IVF/ICSI, with a generally accepted range of 10-20% per cycle for all etiologies [20]. In the literature, the overall pregnancy rate varies from 5% to 30% [3,15]. According to data from the European Society of Human Reproduction and Embryology (ESHRE 2009), the success of IUI in terms of pregnancy rate per cycle varies but could reach 16.4% [21]. In 2018, data from the French biomedicine agency concluded that the average pregnancy rate per cycle of intrauterine insemination with spousal sperm was around 12.4% for that year, with wide variations from one centre to another [5]. Several clinical-biological prognostic factors for both men and women have been reported in relation to IUI results. These factors are related to the type of ovarian stimulation and to the specific characteristics of the couple, such as the woman's age, the type and duration of infertility, the number of mature follicles recruited, the thickness of the endometrium, the number of progressive motile spermatozoa, the morphology of the spermatozoa, the number of motile spermatozoa inseminated, IMC and smoking [14]. However, the predictive value of these parameters remains highly contradictory [22]. The aim of this study was to determine the factors predictive of success in IAC, and to do this we carried out a retrospective study of 328 IUI cycles with spousal sperm in 196 couples.

1. Analytical and correlative study

1.1. Overall results :

In our study, the pregnancy rate was 15.24%, close to that published by some authors [10,22]. In fact, there is considerable variability in the published results regarding the clinical pregnancy rate per cycle of IAC. This variability could be explained by the heterogeneity of the populations treated, the nature of the drugs used, the lack of standard criteria for semen analysis and the different insemination methods or protocols used (Table XIX).

Table XIX: Clinical pregnancy rates per insemination cycle in the literature

Author	Year	Number of cycles	Nature of the study	Study location	Pregnancy rate (%)
Anes et al [23]	2009	522	Retrospective	Tunisia	15,7
Luco et al [14]	2014	356	Retrospective		5,3
Lemmens et al [24]	2016	4251	Retrospective	Neerlandaise	28,2
Thijssen et al [25]	2017	1401	Foresight	Belgium	9,5
Ejzenberg [26]	2019	355	Retrospective	Brazil	15,8
Michau [27]	2019	4146	Retrospective	France	11,5
Hansen [28]	2020	2462	Retrospective	France	14,7
Immediata [29]	2020	7359	Retrospective	Italy	21,89
Our study	2020	328	Retrospective	Tunisia	15,24

1.2.Results based on female parameters:
1.2.1. Age of the woman :
Several published studies have pointed out the importance of a woman's age in all natural and artificial reproduction techniques, and the age-related decline in female fecundity has been well documented, particularly in women undergoing IUI [30-32]. Ferraretti et al in a large retrospective study published in 2017 analysing data from the first 15 years of MAP activity in Europe (19972011), using figures from ESHRE annual reports, noted that in the 1281,203 IUI cycles with spousal sperm, the mean pregnancy and birth rates per cycle were 12.4% and 9.2% in women < 40 years and 8.2% and 4.4% in women > 40 years respectively [33].

Several thresholds have been proposed in these studies to define which patient population benefits most from IUI, and the most frequently found are 35 years.

[34,[35]   38 years [27] 40 years [10,36-41] and 42 years [42]. Stone et al, in a study of 9963 cycles, concluded that the pregnancy rate decreased when the woman's age exceeded 32 years [43]. In a prospective multicentre study, Monraison et al found that the pregnancy rate was 25% in women aged under 27 and 12% in women aged over 39 [8]. Data from European registries at the ESHRE in 2012 showed that the rate of births associated with IUU with spousal sperm decreased with age, i.e. 8.2% under the age of 40 compared with 4.1% over the age of 40 [3]. More recently, Vargas-Tominaga et al, in a retrospective study of 1053 cycles, were able to detect a lower pregnancy rate after the age of 40 compared with patients aged 35 to 39 (2.3% vs 8.9% p<0.05) [44]. This age-related decrease in IUI success rate was explained by these authors as probably due to a combination of factors such as progressive follicular exhaustion, decreased granulosa function, poor oocyte quality [45], decreased endometrial receptivity [32], higher rate of chromosomal abnormalities, increased anovulatory cycles after the age of 40 [31] and immune cell senescence [33].

However, some studies have found that older age had no negative effect on IUI success [46-50]. These differences in results could be explained by the young population in certain studies, such as the study by Ejzenberg et al where the age limit for patients was 38 years [26]. Similarly, in the prospective study by Erdem et al in 2016 including 530 cycles, the mean age of patients was 29.8±5.4 years [51].

In our study we excluded women aged over 40 and divided patients into four age groups: under 30, between 30 and 35, between 35 and 38 and over 38. Pregnancy rates per cycle decreased with age: 15.3% versus 16.5%, 15.6% and 9.1% respectively, but this difference was not significant (p=0.755). In our study population, only 10.1% of women were over 38 years of age and the average age was less than 40 years (32.89±4.29 years).

1.2.2. Hormone levels :
Several studies carried out by different authors have supported the idea that high levels of FSH and estradiol reduce the number of follicles and affect oocyte quality, and therefore present an unfavourable prognostic factor for the treatment of infertility [52-54].

Merviel et al in a retrospective study of 1038 cycles found no significant difference in pregnancy rate with FSH value [10] The same conclusion was reported by Mullin el al (2005) [55]. However, Soria el al found that women with basal FSH <9 IU/L were 3.17 times more likely to become pregnant after IUI than women with basal FSH >9 IU/L [55]. Similarly, Dinelli et al observed a significant decrease in pregnancy rates when FSH levels were >7 IU/L [22]. A recent retrospective study published in 2020 by Immediata et al also confirmed this conclusion [29].

In line with these studies, the pregnancy rate per cycle in our study fell from 21.7% to 9.1% when the FSH level was less than or equal to 7 and >7IU/l respectively. The difference was statistically significant (**p=0.016**) (Table XX).

Table XX: Pregnancy rates and FSH in the literature

Author	Number of IAC cycles	Significance	FSH threshold value
Mullin et al 2005 [55]	1875	0.36	-
Merviel et al 2010 [10]	1038	>0,05	9,4
Soria et al 2012 [56]	3012	**0.008**	**9**
Boulard et al 2013 [57]	535	0,96	
Yavuz et al 2013 [58]	980	**0.004**	**9,4**
Dinelli et al 2014 [22]	2019	**0,021**	7
Bakas et al 2015 [59]	195	>0.05	
Immediata et al 2019 [29]	7359	**< 0.001**	-
Ejzenberg et al 2019 [26]	355	**<0.001**	**7.7**
Anes et al [23]	522	0,1	-
Our study	328	**0,016**	**7**

The impact of the initial LH value at D3 of the cycle on IUI outcomes has been little studied in the literature. Bakas et al noted that the LH level was significantly lower in patients with a clinical pregnancy after 3 cycles of IUI compared with those who had no pregnancy [59]. We found no association between this parameter and the pregnancy rate per IUI cycle (p=0.936).

Boulard et al in a retrospective study of 535 IUI cycles with donor sperm showed that the estradiol level at D3 of the cycle was significantly related to the occurrence of pregnancy (p=0.003) when it was less than 80 pg/ml with a probability of success of 19% [57]. On the other hand, several authors found no significant association between pregnancy rate and basal estradiol level in IUI cycles with spousal sperm [10,55,60] (Table XXI).

In our study, the level of estradiol did not have an impact on IUI results, which could be explained by the fact that the number of IUI cycles with a high level of restradiol >80pg/ml was small (n=9).

Table XXI: Correlation between pregnancy rate per TCI cycle and estradiol

Authors	Year	Number of cycles	p-value	Estradiol level (pg/ml)
Mullin et al [55]	2005	1875	0,28	
Merviel et al [10]	2010	1038	**0,05**	
Lamazou et al [61]	2011	316	>0,05	
Boulard et al [57]	2013	535	**0,04**	80
Bakas et al 2015 [59]	2015		>0.05	
Moro et al [60]	2016	276	0.195	
Dondik et al [62]	2017	209	0.986	
Ejzenberg et al [26]	2019	355	0.773	
Our study	2021	328	0,511	89

AMH is known as a quantitative marker of ovarian reserve and is considered to be the first marker to decrease in the event of a fall in ovarian reserve. It is a reliable marker of ovarian reserve with the ability to predict poor response to multi-follicular stimulation [63].

In a study by Lamazou et al including 316 couples (2944 cycles) with cervical or idiopathic infertility undergoing their first insemination and divided into three different groups according to their AMH levels (<1ng/ml, between 1 and 4.5 ng/ml and >4.5ng/ml). No significant difference was noted in terms of pregnancy rate between these different groups, i.e. 15.5%, 15.2% and 13.5% respectively [61]. Dosso et al confirmed these findings in a retrospective study of 571 women, showing that unlike IVF, an AMH level <1.7ng/ml did not influence the chances of pregnancy in IUI (p=0.5) [64].

However, in another retrospective study of Greek populations, published in 2017, the authors assessed the usefulness of AMH in predicting clinical pregnancy following IUI and compared it with other markers of ovarian reserve (antral follicle count (AFC) and basal FSH assay), They showed that the mean AMH level was significantly higher in the pregnant group than in the non-pregnant group (2.775 ng/ml vs 1.5ng/ml) (p=0.0004) but AMH alone did not have a better predictive value than the other markers of ovarian reserve studied in these patients [62]. Moro et al in 2016 evaluated a population of couples with only unexplained infertility undergoing their first insemination and found that serum AMH was a better marker than CFA for predicting pregnancy outcome after IUI [60]. Michau et al in a recent study published in 2019 showed that a fall in ovarian reserve with an AMH level < 1 ng/ml significantly reduced the chances of clinical pregnancy in IUI (12.5% if AMH > 1 ng/m vs 8.5% if AMH < 1 ng/ml, p=0.01) [27]. These differences in results have been explained by certain authors [65] by the fact that ovarian reserve was closely correlated with age, making it difficult to differentiate the effect of age and ovarian reserve on pregnancy rates. In a retrospective study of 509 couples in different groups according to age and AMH levels and undergoing a maximum of 4 IUI attempts, they showed that the specific AMH levels in each of these couples were significantly different from those in the other groups, that age-specific AMH levels have only a slight effect on IUI results (not significant) when adapting the doses of FSH used [65] (Table XXII).

In our study, we divided our patients into three groups according to AMH levels: <1ng/ml, between 1 and 4.5 ng/ml and >4.5 ng/ml, with pregnancy rates of 12.1%, 27.1% and 16.7% respectively. There was a lower pregnancy rate when AMH was <1ng/ml compared with the other groups but this difference was not significant (p=0.109). This could be explained by the high number of patients with an AMH >1ng/ml (84.1% of cases).

Table XXII: Correlation between pregnancy rate and AMH in the literature

Author	Year	Place of study	Number of cycles	P value	AMH threshold (ng/ml)
Tremellen et al [66]	2010	Australia	1032	0.30	-
Lamazou et al [61]	2012	France	2944	**<0,0001**	-
Bakas et al [59]	2015	USA	195	**<0.001**	**2,3**
Dosso et al [64]	2015	France	2011	0,5	-
Moro et al [60]	2016	Italy	276	**<0.001**	**2,3**
Dondik et al	2017	Greece	209	**0.0004**	-

[62]					
Michau et al [27]	2019	France	4146	**0.01**	**1**
Our study	2020	Tunisia	328	0,109	-

1.3. Results based on male parameters:

1.3.1. Sperm parameters :

The sperm parameters most frequently studied were the number of progressive motile spermatozoa inseminated after preparation, sperm morphology, the total number of progressive motile spermatozoa in the initial state before sperm preparation, and progressive and total motility. Several studies supported the concept of threshold values for sperm parameters below which IUI becomes significantly less effective.

1.3.1.1. Progressive and total mobility initially and after preparation:

With regard to mobility as defined by the World Health Organisation (WHO), some authors have found a significant impact of progressive "a + b" mobility, total initial "a + b + c" mobility, or progressive and total sperm mobility after preparation [67].

Yavuz et al in a retrospective study published in 2013 noted that 40 pregnancies were obtained when progressive mobility was >50% compared to only 6 pregnancies if progressive mobility was <50%. This difference was statically significant (p=0.001) [58]. Ombelet el al in 2014 in a metanalysis of 55 studies concluded that a threshold value of 30% mobility found in three articles out of six in which mobility was found to be a good predictor of success [12] (Table XXIII).

Consistent with these findings, we found a statically significant difference in initial total and progressive mobility. Pregnancy rates were 11.8% when total mobility was <40% versus 50% when total mobility exceeded 60% (p=0.001). Pregnancy rates were 11.5% if initial progressive mobility was <30% versus 17% and 35.1% if initial progressive mobility was between 30 and 40% and >40% respectively (**p=0.001**). There was no significant association between total and progressive mobility after preparation.

Table XXIII: Progressive or total mobility thresholds determined by previous studies and our study

Author	Year	Study	Number of cycles	Mobility	Impact	Mobility threshold
Dickey et al [40]	1999	Retrospective	4056	Progressive mobility	**Yes***	30%
Muontanaro Gauci et al [68]	2002	Retrospective	495	Total mobility	**Yes***	50%
Lee et al [69]	2002	Retrospective	2846	Total mobility	Yes*	30%
Zhao et al [70]	2004	Retrospective	1007	Total mobility	Yes*	>80%
Yalti et al [71]	2004	Retrospective	268	Total mobility	Yes*	30%
Haim et al [72]	2009	Foresight	248	Mobility 'a	Yes*	10%
Ombelet et al [12]	2014	Meta na lyse	55 studies	Total mobility	Yes*	30%
Jellad et al [73]	2014	Retrospective	223	Mobility 'a	Yes*	10%
Kdous et al [74]	2015	Foresight	295	Progressive mobility	No	-
Mollahmadi et al [75]	2019	Retrospective	350 couples	Non precise	Yes***	-
Ejzenberg et al [26]	2019	Retrospective	355	Progressive mobility	Yes**	35%
Ainsworth et	2020	Retrospective	2912	Non precise	Yes***	-

al[76]

| Our study | 2021 | Retrospective | 328 | Total mobility
Progressive mobility | Yes* | 40%
40% |

*Before preparation**After preparation***Before and after preparation

1.3.1.2. Initial total progressive motile sperm count (TPMSC) :

Mankus et al attempted to clarify the relationship between the total number of progressive motile spermatozoa before preparation and live birth rates in couples who had benefited from IUI cycles. In their study including 310 women and 655 cycles, no relationship was detected between initial PMSC and live birth rates. There were no live births with a count <2 million [77]. Similarly, in a retrospective study, Lemmens et al included 1166 couples undergoing 4251 cycles of IUI and showed that the initial MSCWR had no prognostic value in predicting pregnancies in IUI cycles [24].

Our results are in line with the literature and we did not find a significant association between the initial MSCWT rate and pregnancy rates after IUI: the highest pregnancy rate was obtained after >20 million MSCWT (14 pregnancies) whereas only 8 pregnancies were obtained when the MSCWT was between 10 and 15 million but this difference was not significant between the different groups (p=0.304).

1.3.1.3. Number of inseminated progressive motile spermatozoa NSMPI :

In the literature, the NSMPI thresholds recommended for IUI varied considerably from 1 million [22], 5 million [78] and 10 million [79] for patients of any age.

In 2004, a meta-analysis of 16 studies evaluating the results of NSMPI and IUI concluded that at thresholds between 0.8 and 5 million, the specificity of NSMPI, defined as the ability to predict pregnancy failure, was as high as 100%; and the sensitivity of the test, defined as the ability to predict pregnancy, was limited [80].

Ombelet et al published in 2014 a review of 24 articles in which NSMPI was cited as an important predictive parameter: in seven studies a cut-off value of 1 million was mentioned, a cut-off value between 1 and 2 million was used in four studies and other authors mentioned a cut-off value of 5 million [12].

In a retrospective study including 737 couples receiving 2062 cycles for heterogenous indications, Gubert et al studied the impact of different levels of NSMPI according to female age. The results suggested that NSMPI could be used as a predictor of IUI success in women aged <35 years; these women should be informed of their low pregnancy rate when NSMPI is <5 million. In patients over 35, NSMPI did not appear to be a useful predictor of success [81]. Although this study only considered two age categories (<35 years and >35 years), this finding was consistent with other studies in that NSMP I was not a useful predictor of success in older patients [34,82].

In 2021, in a large study published including 92471 cycles in 37553 couples, Muthigi et al attempted to clarify the relationship between sperm concentration and pregnancy rate after IUI; it appeared that the total motile sperm count after preparation was significantly correlated with pregnancy rate when it was below 9 million but was no longer correlated with pregnancy rate above 9 million. As the relationship was continuous and gradual, it was not reasonable to consider this threshold to indicate or not to indicate IUI, but it was useful to use this threshold to establish a prognosis of success and to specify the action to be taken [83].

Another recent prospective multicentre study of 2462 couples with unexplained infertility showed that a higher NSMPI was associated with a higher live birth rate of 14.8% for 15.1 to 20.0 million versus 5.5% when the NSMPI was <5 million [28]. However, live births occurred with an NSMPI <1 million (5.1%). Above an NSMPI of 20 million, the live birth rate per IUI did not increase. The authors concluded that the live birth rate after IUI with NSMPI <1 million was similar to that of IUI seen with NSMPI >1-5 million. This study suggests that there may be no threshold below which live birth is not possible with IUI [28].

In a meta-analysis published in 2020 by Starosta et al encompassing a total of 220 articles of which 102 were selected, the authors found that most of the data supported IUI in couples with an initial TPMSC > 5 million and NSMPI > 1 million [84].

However, Immediata et al, in their studies published in 2020 including 7359 cycles, did not find an impact of NSMPI on pregnancy rates in infertile couples who had undergone IUI [29], in agreement with Hassan et al [85] (Table XXIV).

NSMPI may have unique prognostic value because it reflects both sperm concentration and progressive mobility, as well as the effects of sperm processing [80] .

In this study, patients with NSMPI <1 million were excluded. We found a statically significant decrease in the pregnancy rate per cycle in the NSMPI <5 million group compared with the NSMPI >5 million group, i.e. 5.3% vs 17.9% (p=0.007). To refine our results, we separated IUI cycles into 4 groups according to NSMPI value: <5 million; 5-10 million; 10-15 million; 15-20 million and >20 million. The pregnancy rates were 5.3%, 8.7%, 16.9%, 26.5% and 26.7% respectively. The difference between these different groups was statically significant (p=0.001).

Most authors have studied the minimum number of spermatozoa available for IUI, although no data on the maximum number of inseminated progressive motile spermatozoa has been published. A study published recently in 2021 aimed to determine whether there is a maximum threshold for NSMPI during IUI, above which the live birth rate is adversely affected. In this latest study, Delaroche et al included 2592 IUI cycles in women aged <38 years, with NSMPI >1 million. Live birth rates were 17.9% if 10<NSMPI<20 million, and 22.7% if 20<NSMPI<30 million. The authors concluded that the live birth rate after IUI can be optimised by inseminating a maximum of 30 million motile spermatozoa. They considered that IUI preparations should not be diluted when more than 10 million motile spermatozoa are obtained [86]. In our study, the maximum insemination threshold proposed was 20 million NSMPI. In fact, we found no significant difference if the NSMPI was between 15.1 and 20 million or >20 million, i.e. a pregnancy rate of 26.5% vs 25.7% respectively (p=0.812). This result was consistent with that of Hansen et al who also found that above an NSMPI of 20 million, the live birth rate per IUI does not increase [9].

Table XXIV: NSMPI thresholds recommended by the literature and our study

Author	Year	Study	Number of cycles	Impact	Minimum threshold (millions)
Ombelet [87]	1997	Retrospective	792	Yes	1
Cohlen et al [88]	2000	Metanalysis	3662	Yes	1
Van Weert [80]	2004	Metanalysis	16 studies	Yes	0,8-5
Wainer [78]	2004	Retrospective	2564	Yes	5
Tomlinson [89]	2013			Yes	5
Ombelet	2014	Metanalysis	24 studies	Yes	1

[12]					1-2 5
Jellad et al [73]	2014	Retrospective	223	Yes	5
Dinelli et al [22]	2014				1
Kdous et al [74]	2015	Foresight	295	Yes	1
Lemmens et al [24]	2016	Retrospective	4251	Yes	5-10
Gubert et al [81]	2019	Retrospective		Yes if female age<35	5
Michau et al [27]	2019	Retrospective	4146	Yes	5
Starosta et al [84]	2020	Review	102 studies	Yes	1
Muthigi et al [83]	2021	Retrospective	92471	Yes if <9million	-
Our study	2021	Retrospective	328	Yes	5

1.3.1.4. Sperm morphology :

The results of studies concerning the impact of morphology on the outcome of IUI are difficult to interpret due to the coexistence of several classification systems, different operating procedures for assessing morphology and different inclusion criteria for subjects. The guide to good clinical practice recommends IUI in the absence of severe teratospermia on the baseline sperm count, with no predefined threshold.

In our laboratory, we use the modified David classification for the evaluation of sperm morphology. The lowest pregnancy rate in our study was observed for a percentage of typical forms (FT)<10% (8.2% vs 24.7% if the percentage of FT was >15%; p=0.001).

Prior to 2011, some studies showed that the pregnancy rate per IUI was higher for a value of typical shapes above a threshold defined as 4% according to strict Kruger criteria [34,69,90-93]. However, other studies have found no significant impact of morphology on pregnancy rate [94]. A meta-analysis including 18 articles, 6 of which analysed threshold values, showed that the impact of sperm morphology on pregnancy rates was significant from a threshold of 4 to 5%, when the strict Kruger criteria were used [91]. In a metanalysis published by Ombelet et al in 2014 including 11 out of 16 studies, typical forms >5% (Kruger criteria) were reported as the best threshold value for predicting IUI outcome [12]. In a prospective study published by Erdem et al in 2016, the percentage of normal forms (before and after preparation) was significantly higher in patients who delivered a live baby, but only in the male infertility subgroup [51]. More recent publications on the subject have found no significant difference in pregnancy rates in IUI cycles between groups with or without isolated teratozoospermia [24,95,96] (Table XXV). In a meta-analysis published in 2017 including 20 studies with 41018 IUI cycles, the authors did not find a significant impact of morphology on pregnancy rates if morphology was >4% or <4% (14.2% versus 12.1%, p = 0.06) and concluded that an isolated abnormality in sperm morphology should not exclude couples from an IUI trial [97]. These conflicting results were probably due to the wide range of intra- and inter-laboratory variations in the assessment of sperm morphology, differences in staining methods, morphological classifications used and characteristics of the population studied, such as duration of infertility, female factors (age, ovarian reserve) and causes of infertility.

Table XXV: Effect of sperm morphology on the outcome of IUI cycles according to the literature and our study

Author	Year	Location	Study	Number of cycles	Classification morphological	Impact	Threshold (FT)
Wainer et al [78]	2004	France	Retrospective	2564	David	Yes**	30%
Badawy et al [34]	2009	Egypt	Foresight	714	David	Yes**	30% (Si NSMPI>5 million)
Merviel et al [10]	2010	France	Retrospective	1038	David	Yes*	30%
Jellad et al [73]	2014	Tunisia	Retrospective	223	David modifies	Yes*	20%
Deveneau [96]	2014	United States	Retrospective	856	Kruger	Yes*	4%
Kdous et al[74]	2015	Tunisia	Foresight	295	David modifies	Yes*	20%
Erdem et al [51]	2016	Turkish	Foresight	530	Kruger	Yes***	4.5% (In the male infertility sub-group)
Lemmens [24]	2016	France	Retrospective	2564	Kruger	Yes*	4%
Thijssen et al[25]	2017	Belgium	Foresight	1401	Kruger	No*	
Ejzenberg [26]	2019	Brazil	Retrospective	355	Kruger	Yes**	4%
Our study	2020	Tunis	Retrospective	328	David modifies	Yes	15%

*Before preparation**After preparation***Before and after preparation

1.3.2. Tobacco :

In order to identify possible associations between smoking and male infertility, numerous studies have been conducted, with some reporting contradictory results. While many studies have reported a negative impact of smoking on sperm parameters and male fertility [98,99], others have found no such effect [100,101]. Furthermore, even studies reporting an effect of smoking on sperm parameters have not clearly demonstrated an effect of smoking on male fertility [102,103]. Few authors have studied this factor in IUI. Thijssen et al showed that smoking had a significant negative effect on pregnancy rate in cases where the partner smoked 1 to 14 cigarettes per day compared with non-smokers (P = 0.0165) [25].

In our study, we found no association between smoking and pregnancy rates after IUI (p=0.637). Our results are consistent with those of Dupuis et al and Merviel et al who also found no significant impact of this parameter on IUI outcomes [10,108].

1.4. Results as a function of the parameters relating to the two members of the couple :

1.4.1. Duration of infertility :

Lengthening the duration of infertility appears to be a negative predictive factor for pregnancy after IUI according to the majority of authors [47,48,50,104]. Steures et al attributed a negative coefficient of -0.03 per year of infertility. The precise limits of the duration of infertility for recommending IUI have not been clearly established [105]. Nuojua-Huttunen et al reported a significant difference in pregnancy rates after IUI depending on whether the duration of infertility was < or > 6 years (14.2% versus 6.1%) [36]. Iberico and Houmard reported a decrease in pregnancy rate per cycle from 10.6% to 7.1% for the former and from 9% to 2.2% for the latter depending on whether infertility lasted less or more than 3 years [41,48]. Other authors have shown that infertility lasting less than 5 years is a favourable factor for IUI [35,106]. Cao et al showed that the pregnancy rate decreased significantly if the duration of infertility was >4 years: 16.58% if the duration of infertility was <4 years compared with 8.27% if the duration of infertility was >4 years, p=0.000 [107]. In a second study with a randomised trial, Hansen et al confirmed that the duration of infertility was a predictive factor of IUI success in couples with unexplained infertility [9].

In line with these findings, in our study we noted the absence of pregnancy in couples with a duration of infertility >6 years. A negative and significant association was noted between the duration of infertility and the pregnancy rate per cycle. This rate fell from 19.3% when the duration of infertility was < years to 12% when the duration of infertility was between 3 and 5 years (p=0.02).

However, for other authors, the success rate appears to be little or not influenced by the duration of infertility [8,10,17,22,108].

1.4.2. Type of infertility :

In our study, women with secondary infertility had higher pregnancy rates than women with primary infertility (17.1% vs 14.1%) but this difference was not statistically significant (p=0.475). Several authors found no significant association between the type of infertility and the pregnancy rate after IUI [10,26,36,105]. On the other hand, Dinelli et al analysing 2019 cycles in a retrospective study considered that secondary infertility was a positive prognostic factor (pregnancy rate 16.7% if the infertility was secondary vs 13.7% if the infertility was primary; p=0.04) [22].

1.4.3. Indications for IUI :

After 36 years since the first randomised controlled trial by Kerin at al in 1984 [109], the indications for IUI remain a subject of debate today. Although some authors consider ovulatory problems and mild sperm abnormalities to be among the best indications for IUI, idiopathic infertility remains the most frequent indication [6]. Idiopathic or unexplained infertility represented 44.2% of the causes of infertility in our study, followed by male hypofertility (27.4%). The results of our study were comparable to those found in the literature (table XXVI).

Table XXVI our study	Repartition of the origins of infertility in the literature and in the medical literature.				
Author	Number of cycles	Infertility unexplained	Hypofertilite male	Origin women	Infertility Mixed
Merviel 2010 [10]	1038	10.5%	**32.6%**	24.3%	32.6%
Dinelli et al 2014 [22]	2019	10.9%	**25,8%**	31%	24.0%
Fauque 2017[15]	862	32.5%	19,9%	**47,6%**	-
Cabry- Goubet 2017 [110]	1251	**36%**	12%		
Monraisin et al 2016 [8]	1827	**39 %**	12%	19%	11%

Haller et al 2017 [111]	1092	**46 %**	12 %	25%	
Sicchieri 2018 [112]	237	**25.**32%	16.46%		
Michau 2019 [27]	4146	33%	20,8%	**41,1%**	4,8%
Moreau 2019 [65]	2063	**49,5%**	11,6%	36	2,9%
Ejzenberg 2019 [26]	355	18.0%	15.2%	**32,4%**	27.9%
Immediata el al 2020 [29]	6323	**53.55%**	19.69%	10.95%	
Our 2021 study	328	**44,2%**	27,4%	18,9	9,5%

Polycystic ovary syndrome was diagnosed by the presence of at least 2 of the following 3 criteria: oligo-anovulation, clinical and/or biological hyperandrogenism and/or ultrasound evidence of polycystic ovaries, using the Rotterdam 2003 criteria [113]. The management of anovulation in a patient with PCOS has followed a well-codified strategy since the Thessaloniki Consensus Conference published in 2008 [114]. The first-line treatment is based on ovulation stimulation with clomiphene citrate. When women are said to be "resistant to clomiphene citrate", the choice is between ovarian drilling and ovarian stimulation with gonadotropins [114].

Merviel et al and Soria et al concluded in their studies that the highest pregnancy rates were obtained in patients with PCOS [10,56]. Dinelli et al also obtained the highest pregnancy rate in the PCOS group, 25.4% compared with 13.2% and 15.8% in the unexplained infertility and male hypofertility groups respectively [22].

The risks of ovarian stimulation in these women are OHH and multiple pregnancies [115].

In our study, 75.7% of patients with PCOS were stimulated with gonadotropins and only two patients had undergone ovarian drilling. In agreement with the results of the literature, we observed a higher pregnancy rate in patients with PCOS (35.1%), of whom 2 patients (5.7%) had multiple pregnancies. We did not observe ovarian hyperstimulation syndrome in these patients.

Unexplained infertility was defined by normal ovarian reserve, pelvic ultrasound, hysterosalpingography, spermogram and adequate frequency of intercourse. Unexplained infertility has been diagnosed in up to 30% of couples presenting with infertility [116]. In 2013, NICE (National Institute of Health and clinical Excellence) stated that IUI was not recommended in couples with unexplained infertility, male hypofertility and mild endometriosis, unless the couples had religious, cultural or social characteristics that objected to IVF [117]. However, not all practising clinicians clearly shared the conclusions drawn by NICE. Nandi et al conducted an online survey of specialist opinions on first-line options in the management of unexplained hypofertility. Only 16% would offer IVF as the recommended first choice of treatment [118]. This confirmed the existence of persistent clinical uncertainty despite published guidelines. In 2015, Kim, Child and Farquhar published an online questionnaire survey of UK fertility clinics and showed that of the 46 clinics that responded, 96% (44/46) continued to offer IUI for unexplained infertility [16]. The most commonly used drugs for ovarian stimulation were gonadotropins (95%), followed by clomiphene citrate (49%) and letrozole (19%) [16]. The recent TUI study presented at ESHRE 2018, which consisted of a randomised controlled trial comparing 3 cycles of IUI with ovarian stimulation and 3 months of waiting (expectant) for couples with unexplained infertility, showed that the live birth rate increased threefold in women treated with IUI (31% versus 9%, p<0.001) [119].

Unexplained infertility was the most frequent indication in our study series (44.2%). The pregnancy rate was 14.5%.

Published studies have shown that, in the case of male causes and in particular moderate or slight alteration of sperm parameters, there was insufficient evidence to recommend or not to recommend IUI in this indication [120]. Others, on the other hand, have shown that IUI is not inferior to IVF in mild male infertility by defining an NSMPI of 3 to 10 million, taking into account the small number of couples included in the study (10% of the total number of couples) [121]. In our study 90 IUI were performed for male infertility, i.e. 27.4% of all indications. 11 clinical pregnancies were obtained, i.e. 12.2%.

In a retrospective study including 1880 IUI cycles, Cochet et al showed a dramatic decrease in the clinical pregnancy rate and live birth rate when patients had a single tube, suggesting that IVF should be the preferred treatment in these cases [122]. Similar results were reported by Berker et al with a reduction in pregnancy rate from 44.7% in controls to 26.3% in cases of unilateral tubal obstruction [123]. Several authors suggest that these patients with tubal pathologies should switch to IVF after two cycles of IUI because of the low pregnancy rates [84]. However, other authors have found no difference in pregnancy rate whatever the condition of the tube [124,125].

In our study, tubal pathology accounted for 5.3% of indications. The pregnancy rate in patients with tubal infertility was lower at 10.5%.

The recommendations for clinical practice issued by the CNGOF and endorsed by the French National Authority for Health (HAS) suggested that IUI should only be considered in cases of minimal to mild endometriosis [126]. In a recent review of 2020, Cosma et al, proposed 9 classes of endometriosis and according to them, IUI can be proposed in cases of endometriosis class C3 (C: subfertile patient with an early stage of endometriosis) with absence of spontaneous pregnancy 6 months after surgery in cases of stage 1 /2 ASRM; the pregnancy rate in this group was similar to unexplained infertility [127]. For stage 1-2 endometriosis, pregnancy rates per IUI cycle ranged from 5.2% to 6.5% [84].

In their study Van der Houwen et al, suggested a benefit in pregnancy rate with the use of GnRH agonist during IUI in patients with moderate to severe endometriosis. However, the retrospective nature of the study, the small number of patients, and the absence of data on stimulation limited the validity of these results [128]. Merviel et al obtained a low pregnancy rate of 10.7% in patients with stage 1 or 2 endometriosis [10].

In our study, stage 1 and 2 endometriosis accounted for only 3.5% of indications for IUI. No pregnancies were observed in these patients (n=3).

In line with the recent study by Starosta in 2020, in our work IUI was more effective for women with ovulatory dysfunction (35.1%) and unexplained infertility (14.5%), and less effective for women with tubal pathology (10.5%) and stage 1 or 2 endometriosis (0%). The difference in pregnancy rates according to the indications for TIA was statically significant (p=0.024), bearing in mind that the frequency of women suffering from endometriosis and vaginismus was very low (n=3 and n=2 respectively).

1.5. Results as a function of parameters relating to the conduct of TSI cycles :

1.5.1. What treatments are used in stimulated cycles? What are the doses?

IUI combined with ovarian stimulation is proving to be an effective form of treatment for hypofertile couples. Several protocols for ovarian stimulation combined with IUI have been proposed, but which protocol and which dose are the most effective and economical?

Several drugs are available to achieve ovarian hyperstimulation. The oldest is probably CC in doses of 50 to 150 mg per day for 5 days from the start of the cycle. Being an anti-restrogen, you need to be aware of its negative action on the endometrium. This could explain the low pregnancy rates observed with CC compared with other drugs [129]. Furthermore, the use of CC did not prevent the occurrence of multiple pregnancies [130]. CC alone does not appear to have a significant influence on the success rate of IUI [25,46,131,132].

In a 2007 meta-analysis of 43 trials (3957 women), the authors found in 7 randomised controlled trials that the pregnancy rate was higher with gonadotropins than with CC (OR 1.8; 95% CI, 1.2-2.7), regardless of the etiology of infertility [130]. This concept was supported by the M-OVIN trial published in 2018, which involved women with anovulation after six failed cycles of IUI with CC [133]. The live birth rate was better in the gonadotropin-stimulated insemination group than in the CC group, 52% vs 41% respectively [133]. In another multicentre randomised controlled trial comparing gonadotropins with CC in couples with unexplained hypofertility in IUI cycles with strict cancellation criteria, the pregnancy rate was 31% in women treated with gonadotropins and 26% in women treated with CC (relative risk (RR) 1.16, 95% CI 0.93 to 1.47 [134].

Letrozole is a 3rd generation aromatase inhibitor, which can be used alone for simple ovarian stimulation, or in combination with gonadostimulins, and has no antiestrogenic effect on the endometrium or cervical mucus. Ovarian stimulation with letrozole was first performed by Mitwally and Casper in 2001 after unsuccessful treatment with CC in 22 patients with ovulatory hypofertility. These authors concluded that letrozole was an effective treatment for ovulation induction and increased follicular recruitment in dysovulatory women without adverse effects on the endometrium [135] . In another study, these authors reported reduced gonadotropin requirements and improved pregnancy rates when letrozole was combined with FSH for ovarian stimulation in patients with a history of poor response to stimulation with FSH alone [135].

On the contrary, other authors have found no significant difference when comparing anti-estrogens (CC) with aromatase inhibitors [130]. In a prospective randomised trial including 280 women with unexplained infertility, the authors concluded that the use of CC or letrozole during ovarian stimulation to reduce the dose of gonadotropins was justified and that this approach would reduce the cost of stimulation protocols without any effect on treatment results, and letrozole had no advantage over CC in this respect [136].

In women with PCOS receiving stimulated IUI, CC, letrozole and gonadotropins were all equally effective and safe in the retrospective study by Huang et al published in 2018 where the authors concluded that letrozole had the highest monofollicular growth rate and recommend this drug as the treatment of first choice in infertile women candidates for ovulation induction in IUI cycles [137]. Similarly, in a recent comparative study published in 2020, Nguyen considered that letrozole used to stimulate the ovaries of infertile women with PCOS, combined with intrauterine insemination, is an effective treatment [138].

It should be noted that letrozole has not yet been granted marketing authorisation (MA) in France for this indication, despite recent studies which showed no difference in terms of congenital malformations compared with CC [139].

In a 2018 Cochrane review, Franik analysed 42 randomised controlled trials using letrozole in 7935 women with polycystic ovary syndrome to assess the effectiveness of aromatase inhibitors for these women for ovulation induction, followed by planned intercourse or IUI. These analyses showed a higher rate of live births and pregnancy rates with letrozole than with CC. However, he found no difference in the rates of miscarriage, multiple pregnancy and hyperstimulation syndrome (HSO) [140].

Yun et al 2015 suggested that minima stimulation using gonadotropins every other day with letrozole decreased the development of OHSS and multiple pregnancies, while maintaining comparable pregnancy rates in IUI cycles [141].

In our study, the highest pregnancy rate was obtained after ovarian stimulation with the combination of CC and FSH with 19.3% versus 12.7% and 13.6% after ovarian stimulation with CC+HMG and CC respectively, but the difference was not significant compared with the other molecules used (p=0.469). This may be explained by the heterogeneity of our study population. The use of Letrozole resulted in 50% pregnancies, but this molecule was only used in 2 cases, i.e. 0.6% of the cycles studied. Other authors have described no significant influence of the type of stimulation on pregnancy rates after IUI [22,88,94].

In Cantineau's review, which included 43 studies involving 3957 women, he showed that gonadotropins should be used at a low dose because the rate of multiple pregnancies was increased with high-dose injections, without any increase in pregnancy rates [130]. However, for Ghaffari, the total dose of gonadotropins was positively associated with the outcome of IUI in terms of pregnancy (p=0.03) [108].

In our study, the doses of FSH and HMG had no impact on our results.

1.5.2. Single, partial or multiple follicular stimulation?

In a retrospective study including 1038 cycles, Merviel et al found that a bi-follicular objective was associated with a better chance of pregnancy in IUI: 9.8% of clinical pregnancies per cycle if 1 mature follicle was present on the day of induction versus 14.5% if 2 mature follicles were present (p <0.01) [10]. Soria et al analysed 3012 cycles and confirmed this conclusion [56]. Monra sin et al in a multicentre study showed an increase in delivery rates in IUI cycles when going from 1 to 2 follicles, i.e. 9% versus 16%, p<0.001 [8]. Michau et al also showed a significant difference in terms of clinical pregnancy when going from 1 to 2 follicles, i.e. 11% in monofollicular versus 14.4% in bi-follicular (p=0.01) with an increased risk of twin pregnancies [27]. Recently, Vargas-Tominaga et al in their study published in 2020 concluded that having two or more follicles was the most important predictive factor for successful IUI cycles with a pregnancy rate of 11.6% with > 2 follicles and 4.4% with < 2 follicles [44].

Our study was in agreement with these results; the pregnancy rate rose from 8.6% after monofollicular stimulation to 18.77% when 2 or more follicles were obtained (p=0.015).

However, the risk of multiple pregnancy increased with the number of follicles, especially when three or more follicles were recruited [142]. This finding has been reported in numerous studies [8,10].

The number of follicles was >2 follicles in the three multiple pregnancies obtained in our study.

1.5.3. Thickness of the endometrium :

There is conflicting evidence in the literature regarding endometrial thickness (EE) and pregnancy rates. Several studies have reported significant correlations between pregnancy rates and endometrial thickness [22,143] while others have found no such relationship [133].

Esmailzadeh et al considered that EE could be a major predictor of IUI success and suggested that clinicians providing IUI to infertile couples should pay particular attention to endometrial development as well as follicle growth and sperm mobility [143]. Dinelli et al also found that endometrial thickness had a significant impact on IUI outcome: the highest pregnancy rate was obtained when the EE varied between 10 and 11 mm [22].

In a meta-analysis published in 2017 including 23 studies comprising 3846 women, the authors concluded that EE did not appear to be a predictive factor of success in IUI with ovarian stimulation and suggested that it might be desirable to examine other biomarkers. It was suggested that subendometrial neovascularisation measured by three-dimensional Doppler ultrasound may predict pregnancy in women undergoing IUI. They concluded that cancellation of IUI cycles due to thin endometrial mucosa may have a negative impact on clinical care [133].

Danhof et al proposed that the difference in pregnancy rate between gonadotropin stimulation and CC could be explained by a difference in endometrial thickness, these authors performed a second analysis of data from a metanalysis published in 2018 including patients with unexplained infertility who had undergone IUI and found that gonadotropin use resulted in a thicker endometrium than clomiphene citrate [134]. However, in a review published in 2020, the difference in endometrial thickness did not affect the pregnancy rate. Therefore, for these authors, a relatively thin endometrium after clomiphene citrate was not a reason to prefer gonadotropins as the best molecule for stimulation in cases of unexplained hypofertility [144].

Our results are consistent with the literature: we found a statically significant association between pregnancy rate and endometrial thickness, with a mean of 9.7±1.5 mm in patients who had become pregnant compared with 8.48±1.7 mm in the group of non-pregnant patients (p=0.000), and the pregnancy rate was 17.4% in the group of women with EE <9 mm compared with 40.6% if the EE was >9 mm (p=0.001).

1.5.4. The ideal time for insemination :

The survival of spermatozoa in the upper part of the female genital tract is patent, hence the need for precise timing between IUI and ovulation [111]. The timing of insemination was considered to be one of the most important factors influencing the results of IUI. There were several methods of timing IUI, of which LH measurement (in natural cycles) or ultrasound monitoring of follicular growth combined with HCG injection were the most widely used [145]. Randomised trials have not found significant differences in clinical pregnancy or live birth rates between different times 24 to 48 hours after HCG injection [146,147]. A recent study found that IUI can be performed between 24 and 40 hours after HCG injection without compromising pregnancy rates [145].

A single prospective randomised study compared pregnancy rates between simultaneous insemination with HCG administration and after 34-36 hours of HCG administration, but the authors found no statistically significant difference with pregnancy rates of 9.4% and 12.2% respectively (p=0.523) [148] (Table XXVII).

Table XXVII : Ideal time of insemination according to the literature

Author	Year	Location	Type of study	Number of cycles	Insemination window
Claman et al [146]	2004	Canada	Foresight	270	32 to 40 hours
Rahman	2011	India	Foresight	399	36 hours

[147]					
Aydin et al [148]	2013	Turkish	Foresight	220	J0- 34a 36 hours
Haller et al [111]	2017	France	Retrospective	1092	J1-J2
Cohlen et al [145]	2018	Amsterdam	Metanalysis	-	24-48 hours
Lee et al [149]	2018	Korea	Retrospective	411	36-38 hours

Another approach that has been proposed to obtain the right timing is to increase the number of inseminations per cycle from one to two (double insemination), by increasing the number of spermatozoa in the ampulla of the fallopian tube. However, the results are controversial. Ragni et al analysed 449 cycles in 273 couples after ovarian stimulation with clomiphene citrate [150]. Double insemination at 12 and 34 h after HCG resulted in a significantly higher pregnancy rate than a single IUI. In a Cochrane review that included two trials, no advantage was shown for double IUI compared with single IUI [130]. This result was confirmed by another larger study, which also showed that double insemination did not provide better pregnancy outcomes than single insemination [151].

In our study, all couples underwent simple insemination 36 to 40 hours after HCG injection.

1.5.5. Sexual abstinence period :

In 2010, the WHO recommended a period of 2 to 7 days of sexual abstinence in its guidelines. Several studies of sperm parameters support this recommendation of 2 to 5 days abstinence, which was associated with significantly higher semen volume and a higher number of progressive motile spermatozoa [152]. In contrast, a recent study reported significantly higher sperm mobility in the ejaculate of infertile men if they were produced within 40 minutes of an initial sample with less than 5 million motile spermatozoa [153]. For some authors, an abstinence period of 0 to 2 days could be accompanied by a higher rate of morphologically normal spermatozoa [152].

Some studies have shown a negative impact of longer abstinence periods on pregnancy rates in cohorts of 372 [152] and 417 couples [154]. These two studies reported higher pregnancy rates in the group with abstinence periods of up to 2 days and up to 3 days respectively [152,154].

In a review of the literature, Lemmens et al recommend changing the WHO recommendation to a maximum abstinence period of 3 days [24].

In our study, we found that in 64% of the 50 pregnancies obtained, the duration of abstinence was <03 days, while in only 2% of pregnancies obtained was the duration >7 days. The highest pregnancy rate (18.3%) was obtained with 4 to 7 days of abstinence. The difference was not statistically significant (p=0.469) (note that the duration of abstinence was >7 days in only 4.3% of IUIs).

1.5.6. Time between sperm preparation and insemination :

In a multicentre study by Fauque et al including 709 patients from 7 different French centres, which aimed to identify the impact of the time interval between the end of sperm preparation and IUI, the authors concluded that an ideal time of 40-80 minutes was necessary to obtain a maximum pregnancy rate [15]. The authors explained this by the fact that when this time was too short, the incubation time required to increase sperm chromatin decondensation was probably insufficient and, on the contrary, when the time was too long, there was a probable negative effect of in vitro environmental conditions and an increase in the spontaneous acrosome reaction rate [15].

In our study, the average time between sperm preparation and the actual insemination procedure was 30 minutes, and there was no significant difference in the clinical pregnancy rate.

1.5.7. Choice of catheter used :

Researchers have suggested that the type of catheter used may influence pregnancy assessment criteria [155]. Several authors have studied the relationship between soft and hard catheters and IUI success. A Cochrane review concluded that there was no evidence of a significant difference in the choice of catheter type for any of the outcome criteria [156].

In our study, a rigid catheter was used to inseminate sperm prepared inside the uterus in only 11% of patients (n=36). The difference between the use of a flexible or rigid catheter was not statistically significant in terms of pregnancy (p=0.293).

1.5.8. Difficult procedure:

Difficult insemination was defined as the occurrence of bleeding during the trial or multiple attempts to perform the IUI.

In a retrospective study, Khan et al showed no difference in the clinical pregnancy rate for easy or difficult IUI [157]. Whereas Vargas et al found that the difficulty of the IUI procedure decreased the pregnancy rate [44].

In our study, the difficulty of insemination had no impact on IUI results (p=0.324).

1.5.9. Support for the luteal phase :

The luteal phase is an important phase of the menstrual cycle during which embryo implantation occurs. A good quality luteal phase is characterised by adequate secretion of progesterone by the corpus luteum and secretory transformation of the endometrium. Support of the luteal phase is necessary in IVF [158] . However, it remains debatable in IUI [13].

Some authors have mentioned that in the case of a spontaneous cycle or with simple stimulation (with 1 or 2 follicles), there was no biological or empirical evidence that treatment with HCG or progesterone during the luteal phase was necessary or improved the pregnancy rate [150]. Similarly, others found no supportive effect of the luteal phase, regardless of the ovarian stimulation protocol used [8].

On the contrary, other authors who compared the different means of luteal support in 26198 women included in 94 randomised controlled studies concluded that HCG or progesterone administered during the luteal phase could be associated with higher rates of live births or clinical pregnancies [159].

Erdem et al studied the efficacy of luteal support using a progesterone gel (Crinine) in IUI cycles stimulated with recombinant gonadotropins in a population with unexplained infertility. The rates of live births per cycle were significantly higher in patients who had vaginal progesterone gel for luteal phase support compared with controls: 39.4% versus 23.8% (p=0.01) [50].

In a recent meta-analysis published in 2017, the authors showed an improvement in pregnancy rates and live births for patients who received progesterone support during the luteal phase. This effect was observed only in patients stimulated with gonadotropins and not with CC. The data in this review would suggest a benefit to luteal phase support during ovarian stimulation with gonadotropins for IUI [160].

Today, no reference treatment in this context is recommended [161]. Nevertheless, the addition of progesterone has become established clinical practice even in the absence of solid evidence of efficacy (ESHRE 2009) [21].

1.5.10. Rank of attempt :

The number of IUI cycles per couple is an important factor to discuss when starting treatment.

In the literature, the number of attempts varies from three to six, depending on the authors and their stimulation practices. Several authors recommend IVF after three failed CAI attempts. In the study by Plosker and Amato, out of 48 pregnancies, 43 occurred during the first 3 cycles and only 5 pregnancies occurred after 3 cycles of treatment [37]. Similarly, Nuojua-Huttunen et al noted that the highest pregnancy rate in 811 cycles (18%) was observed during the first cycle and that 97% of all pregnancies resulted from the first 4 cycles of IAC [36]. Aboulghar et al, conducted a prospective study, including 594 patients with unexplained infertility and patients with minimal to mild endometriosis, all couples received one to three cycles of IUI and 91 couples underwent four to six cycles after IUI failure in the first three cycles. In patients who underwent 1 to 3 cycles followed by IVF, the pregnancy rate per cycle was 39.2% compared with 5.6% in patients who underwent up to 6 cycles (P<0.01). These authors concluded that IVF should be considered after failure of 3 stimulated cycles [165]. Merviel et al also noted that more than 80% of clinical pregnancies were obtained during the first three cycles [10].

Furthermore, Cohlen el al in their metanalysis published in 2018 concluded that at least three consecutive IUI cycles should be performed and that there was insufficient evidence to recommend a maximum number of IUI cycles [145].

In line with results published in the literature, the number of attempts in our study correlated significantly and negatively with the pregnancy rate after insemination; 40.8% of pregnancies were obtained after 2 attempts compared with 20.4% and 10.2% after 3 and 4 attempts respectively (p=0.000). No pregnancy was obtained after the 5th attempt in our series.

1.5.11. Post-insemination complications :

It is absolutely essential to define a strategy that will certainly enable the best pregnancy rates to be obtained without inducing an excessive risk associated with ovarian stimulation: ovarian hyperstimulation (OHS) and multiple pregnancies with their consequences.

It has been well established that multiple pregnancies decrease the probability of live birth and increase the risk to both mother and fetus [164,165]. They were associated with maternal morbidity such as preeclampsia, gestational diabetes, and a 50% risk of premature delivery, leading to significant neonatal morbidity and mortality [166]. Cycles should therefore be closely monitored and when more than two to three follicles larger than 15 mm, or when more than 5 follicles larger than 10 mm are seen, secondary preventive measures may be recommended [125], if cycles could be cancelled and couples should be advised to abstain from unprotected sex. As an alternative to cycle cancellation, aspiration of excess follicles at the time of HCG injection or LH surge, or conversion to IVF, could be additional options to reduce the risk of multiple pregnancies [129].

In our study, no ovarian hyperstimulation syndrome was observed. Pregnancy was multiple in 6.1% (n=3 pregnancies) with 2 gemellar pregnancies and one triplet pregnancy terminated at 2 months.

2. Strengths and limitations of our study :

The strengths of our study are :

^ The patient sample is representative, and the size of the sample studied was sufficient to provide statically reliable results.

J We considered non-inclusion and exclusion criteria with reference to the literature in order to avoid bias and increase the value of our study.

^ We have analysed all the parameters studied and analysed in recent publications.

Nevertheless, this study has a number of limitations:

^ The retrospective design of our study, with all its inherent biases.

^ Not all pregnant women were followed through to delivery, which prevented the evaluation of data on pregnancies and newborns; a primary outcome criterion such as live birth would have been more relevant.

2.1.Recommendations and outlook :

IUI is a frequently used MPA technique for the treatment of hypofertility, but its results depend on a number of factors specific to couples and IUI cycles. The optimal treatment strategy should be based on individual patient characteristics.

We believe that our results may be useful for better counselling and selection of couples consulting for hypofertility, thus increasing the success of IUI cycles before opting for another much more expensive and invasive assisted reproduction treatment. Our results show that :

J IUI is more effective in women with PCOS and unexplained infertility and less effective in women with tubal pathology and endometriosis.

J Results are similar when IUI is performed after primary or secondary infertility.

J IUI is not recommended in the first instance in cases of infertility exceeding 6 years.

J Three IIU cycles is the absolute maximum that should be offered.

J Bi-follicular ovarian stimulation seems to improve the chances of pregnancy, but with a modest increase in the rate of gemellar pregnancies.

J The IUI must be cancelled if more than three mature follicles are obtained, due to the high risk of multiple pregnancies.

J The use of low-dose gonadotropins is recommended.

J A number of inseminated final progressive motile spermatozoa >5 million appears to be predictive of success.

J The chances of success are better, and increase when the NSMPI is above 10, between 10 and 15, and between 15.1 and 20 million, without increasing above an NSMPI of 20 million. We therefore recommend diluting the preparations when more than 20 million progressive motile spermatozoa are obtained.

J Initial progressive and total sperm mobility, as well as the percentage of typical forms, appear to be predictive of success in the outcome of IAC cycles. We therefore recommend initial progressive and total sperm mobility > 40%, and a percentage of typical forms exceeding 15%.

Outlook :

We intend to broaden the study population to include a larger number of people, which would give us a clearer idea of the relevance of our results.

5 CONCLUSIONS

Intrauterine insemination (IUI) is a long-established method of medically assisted procreation, widely used as one of the first lines of treatment for infertile couples and recognised as being the simplest and least expensive. However, the success of an IUI programme is multifactorial. Different therapeutic strategies have been evaluated to improve IUI outcomes. However, the results in terms of clinical pregnancies remain disappointing, suggesting a problem of therapeutic indication.

The aim of our study was to evaluate the prognostic factors of success of IUI in couples receiving cycles of IAC to allow a better orientation of the couples, and thus an optimization of the recourse to the intrauterine insemination starting from a retrospective series of 328 IUI in 196 infertile couples, carried out over a period of four years going from January 2016 to January 2020 with the centre of PMA of the principal military hospital of instruction of Tunis.

A successful IAC attempt was defined by the achievement of a clinical pregnancy with evidence of a gestational sac on ultrasound and/or an eHCG level > 1000 IU/l.

All inseminations were performed after ovulation stimulation. The mean age of our patients was 32.8±4.2 years, with extremes ranging from 20 to 40 years. Infertility was primary in 62.5% of cases and secondary in 37.5%. The mean duration of infertility was 3.3 ± 1.9 years, with extremes ranging from 1 to 11 years. CAI was mainly indicated for unexplained infertility (44.2%) and male infertility (27.4%). The mean basal FSH value was 7.2±2.9 IU/ml with extremes ranging from 1.3 to 21 IU/ml. The mean AMH value was 3.1±2.7 ng/ml with extremes ranging from 0.3 to 16 ng/ml. Tubal patency, at least unilateral, was checked in all patients by hysterosalpingography with or without crelioscopy. 67.4% of the men were smokers. Analysis of sperm parameters showed an average initial sperm concentration on the day of insemination of $53.2±52.9x10^6$ /ml and $75±5.6x10^6$ /ml after preparation, an average initial total mobility of 33.8±13 and 75.1±56 after preparation, 69.5% of patients had asthenospermia with an initial progressive mobility <30%. This asthenospermia was severe (<15%) in 10.1% of patients. The mean initial TMSC was 35.6±44 million, the mean percentage of typical forms of spermatozoa (modified David) was 14.25±10.46% with extremes ranging from

2 a 75%. The mean number of inseminated progressive motile spermatozoa (NSMPI) was 16.98±14.3 million, with extremes ranging from 1 to 67.2 million.

The average number of attempts per couple was 1.7 (1 to 6). The majority of our patients (58.2% of couples) had benefited from a single IUI attempt. Gonadotropins (FSH or HMG) were used in combination with clomiphene citrate (CC) in 76.2% of cycles. The mean doses of gonadotropins used were 359.34±174.82 for HMG and 333.1±174.05 for FSH. The mean number of mature follicles obtained on the day of induction in our study population was 1.9, with extremes of 1 to 4 follicles. Ovarian stimulation was monofollicular in only 35% of cases. The mean endometrial thickness was 8.8±1.8 mm, with extremes of 6 to 15 mm.

We obtained 50 pregnancies, i.e. 15.2% of clinical pregnancies, including one extra uterine pregnancy.

According to our results, the overall rate of clinical pregnancy per cycle fell, but not significantly, with increasing age, from 15.3% in women aged under 30 to 9.1% in those aged 38 and over (p=0.381). This result could be explained by the exclusion of women aged over 40 in our study.

The basal FSH level had an impact on the pregnancy rate, which fell from 21.7% when this level was <7IU/ml to 9.1% when FSH was >9 UI/ml (p=0.016). However, the estradiol level on day 3 and the LH level did not influence the results of the IUI.

With regard to AMH, there was a statically significant impact on the pregnancy rate only in women with PCOS. The latter fell from 72.7% when the AMH level was between 1 and 4.5 ng/ml to 26.3% when the AMH level exceeded 4.5 ng/ml (p=0.032) in these women.

The pregnancy rate increased from 11.5% to 35.1% when the initial progressive mobility was <30% and >40% respectively (p=0.001). Initial total mobility also influenced our results, with a pregnancy rate of 11.8% in cases of asthenospermia defined by total mobility <40% and 20% when total mobility was between 40 and 60% (p=0.02).

We observed a statically significant increase in the chances of successful IUU cycles for NSMPI values >5 million, i.e. a pregnancy rate of 17.9% versus 5.3% if the NSMPI is <5 million; p=0.007 with no obvious increase in the clinical pregnancy rate per cycle when the NSMPI exceeded 20 million. This result suggested that IUI preparations might need to be diluted when more than 20 million motile spermatozoa were recovered in the final pellet.

The best clinical pregnancy rates were obtained with typical forms exceeding 15% using the modified David classification, i.e. 24.7% versus 20% and 8.1% when the mean percentage of typical forms was >15%; 10%<FT<15%, and <10% respectively; p=0.001.

IUI was more effective for women with PCOS and unexplained infertility, with a rate of clinical pregnancies per cycle of 35.1% and 14.5% respectively, and less effective for women with tubal factor (10.5%) and type 1 to 2 endometriosis (0%). The difference between the different etiologies was statically significant (p=0.024).

We found that a shorter duration of infertility was significantly associated with a better prognosis, with the pregnancy rate rising from 19.3% when the duration of infertility was <2 years to 12% when it exceeded 3 years (p=0.02).

However, pregnancy rates in women with secondary infertility tended to be higher than in those with primary infertility (17.1% versus 14.1%), although this was not statistically significant (p=0.475).

The number of attempts correlated significantly and negatively with the pregnancy rate after insemination, with 40.8% of pregnancies obtained after 2 attempts compared with 20.4% and 10.2% obtained after 3 and 4 attempts respectively (p=0.000).

The highest pregnancy rate was obtained after ovarian stimulation with CC+FSH (19.3%), but the difference was not significant compared with the other molecules used (p=0.469).

The rate of clinical pregnancies per cycle as a function of the number of follicles >18mm on the day of initiation rose from 8.6% after monofollicular stimulation to 18.77% when two or more follicles were obtained (p=0.015).

There was also a strong positive and significant association between the clinical pregnancy rate of IUIs per cycle and endometrial thickness. The pregnancy rate increased from 17.4% to 40.6% when the endometrium was <9 mm and >9 mm respectively on the day of induction (p=0.001).

At the end of our study, several factors, both clinical and biological, seem to influence the outcome of IUI cycles, but the indications for IUI, the FSH level at D03 of the cycle, the initial progressive spermatic mobility, the percentage of typical forms, the rank of attempts and the number of follicles are the most predictive factors of the success of IUI cycles.

We suggest and recommend the following
- Basal FSH <7IU/ml
- Bilateral tubal permeability on hysterosalpingography.
- Infertility of unexplained origin and in the case of PCOS.
- A period of infertility of less than 3 years.

- Progressive and total initial sperm mobility >40%.
- NSMPI >5 million.
- A dilution of the final pellet obtained for sperm preparation in the case of NSMPI >20 million.
- A percentage of typical forms >15%.
- Paucifollicular stimulation or stimulation with a number of follicles >2 follicles.
- The endometrium is thicker than 9 mm on the day ovulation begins.
- A maximum of 3 IAC attempts.

6 REFERENCES

1.   Zegers Hochschild F, Adamson GD, De Mouzon J, Ishihara O, Mansour R, Nygren K, et al. International committee for monitoring assisted reproductive technology (ICMART) and the world health organization (WHO) revised glossary of ART terminology, 2009. Fertil Steril. 2009;92(5):1520-4.

2.   Inhorn MC, Patrizio P. Infertility around the globe: new thinking on gender, reproductive technologies and global movements in the 21st century. Hum Reprod Update. 2015;21(4):411-26.

3.   Calhaz Jorge C, De Geyter C, Kupka MS, De Mouzon J, Erb K, Mocanu E, et al. Assisted reproductive technology in europe, 2012: results generated from european registers by ESHRE. Hum Reprod. 2016;31(8):1638-52.

4.   De Geyter C, Calhaz Jorge C, Kupka MS, Wyns C, Mocanu E, Motrenko T, et al. ART in europe, 2014: results generated from European registries by ESHRE: the european ivf-monitoring consortium (EIM) for the european society of human reproduction and embryology (ESHRE). Hum Reprod. 2018;33(9):1586-601.

5.   Agence de la biomedecine. Evaluation des résultats des laboratoires d'assistance medicale a la procreation pratiquant l'insemination artificielle intrauterine en France [Online]. 2018 [cited 14/8/2021]; [20 pages]. Available from URL : https://www.agence-biomedecine.fr/IMG/pdf/national_ia_2018.pdf

6.   Yazbeck C. Too many intrauterine inseminations in France. Gynecol Obstet Fertil Senol. 2021;49(4):223-4.

7.   Sahakyan M, Harlow BL, Hornstein MD. Influence of age, diagnosis, and cycle number on pregnancy rates with gonadotropin-induced controlled ovarian hyperstimulation and intrauterine insemination. Fertil Steril. 1999;72(3):500-4.

8.   Monraisin O, Chansel Debordeaux L, Chiron A, Floret S, Cens S, Bourrinet S, et al. Evaluation of intrauterine insemination practices: a 1-year prospective study in seven french assisted reproduction technology centers. Fertil Steril. 2016;105(6):1589-93.

9.   Hansen KR, He AW, Styer AK, Wild RA, Butts S, Engmann L, et al. Predictors of pregnancy and live-birth in couples with unexplained infertility after ovarian stimulation-intrauterine insemination. Fertil Steril. 2016;105(6):1575-83.

10. Merviel P, Heraud MH, Grenier N, Lourdel E, Sanguinet P, Copin H. Predictive factors for pregnancy after intrauterine insemination (IUI): an analysis of 1038 cycles and a review of the literature. Fertil Steril. 2010;93(1):79-88.

11. Park SJ, Alvarez JR, Weiss G, Von Hagen S, Smith D, McGovern PG. Ovulatory status and follicular response predict success of clomiphene citrate-intrauterine insemination. Fertil Steril. 2007;87(5):1102-7.

12. Ombelet W, Dhont N, Thijssen A, Bosmans E, Kruger T. Semen quality and prediction of IUI success in male subfertility: a systematic review. Reprod Biomed Online. 2014;28(3):300-9.

13. Van Der Linden M, Buckingham K, Farquhar C, Kremer JM, Metwally M. Luteal phase support for assisted reproduction cycles. Cochrane Database Syst Rev. 2015 Jul 7;2015(7):CD009154.

14. Luco SM, Agbo C, Behr B, Dahan MH. The evaluation of pre and post processing semen analysis parameters at the time of intrauterine insemination in couples diagnosed with male factor infertility and pregnancy rates based on stimulation agent. A retrospective cohort study. Eur J Obstet Gynecol Reprod Biol. 2014;179:159-62.

15. Fauque P, Lehert P, Lamotte M, Bettahar Lebugle K, Bailly A, Diligent C, et al. Clinical

success of intrauterine insemination cycles is affected by the sperm preparation time. Fertil Steril. 2014;101(6):1618-23.

16. Kim D, Child T, Farquhar C. Intrauterine insemination: a UK survey on the adherence to NICE clinical guidelines by fertility clinics. BMJ Open. 2015;5(5):e007588.

17. Goverde AJ, McDonnell J, Vermeiden JP, Schats R, Rutten FF, Schoemaker J. Intrauterine insemination or in-vitro fertilisation in idiopathic subfertility and male subfertility: a randomised trial and cost-effectiveness analysis. Lancet. 2000;355(9197):13-8.

18. Tjon Kon Fat RI, Bensdorp AJ, Bossuyt PM, Koks C, Oosterhuis GE, Hoek A, et al. Is IVF-served two different ways-more cost-effective than IUI with controlled ovarian hyperstimulation? Hum Reprod. 2015;30(10):2331-9.

19. Ghaffari F, Sadatmahalleh SJ, Akhoond MR, Eftekhari Yazdi P, Zolfaghari Z. Evaluating the effective factors in pregnancy after intrauterine insemination: a retrospective study. Int J Fertil Steril. 2015;9(3):300-8.

20. Duran HE, Morshedi M, Kruger T, Oehninger S. Intrauterine insemination: a systematic review on determinants of success. Hum Reprod Update. 2002;8(4):373- 84.

21. ESHRE Capri Workshop Group. Intrauterine insemination. Hum Reprod Update. 2009;15(3):265-77.

22. Dinelli L, Courbiere B, Achard V, Jouve E, Deveze C, Gnisci A, et al. Prognosis factors of pregnancy after intrauterine insemination with the husband's sperm: conclusions of an analysis of 2,019 cycles. Fertil Steril. 2014;101(4):994-1000.

23. Barberet J, Boucret L, Fauque P, May Panloup P. Assistance medicale a la procreation: techniques actuelles et nouveaux horizons. Rev Francoph Lab. 2018;2018(504):43-51.

24. Lemmens L, Kos S, Beijer C, Brinkman JW, Van Der Horst FL, Van Den Hoven L, et al. Predictive value of sperm morphology and progressively motile sperm count for pregnancy outcomes in intrauterine insemination. Fertil Steril. 2016;105(6):1462 -8.

25. Thijssen A, Creemers A, Van Der Elst W, Creemers E, Vandormael E, Dhont N, et al. Predictive value of different covariates influencing pregnancy rate following intrauterine insemination with homologous semen: a prospective cohort study. Reprod Biomed Online. 2017;34(5):463-72.

26. Ejzenberg D, Gomes TO, Monteleone PA, Serafini PC, Soares JM, Baracat EC. Prognostic factors for pregnancy after intrauterine insemination. Int J Gynaecol Obstet. 2019;147(1):55-72.

27. Michau A, El Hachem H, Galey J, Le Parco S, Perdigao S, Guthauser B, et al. Predictive factors for pregnancy after controlled ovarian stimulation and intrauterine insemination: a retrospective analysis of 4146 cycles. J Gynecol Obstet Hum Reprod. 2019;48(10):811-5.

28. Hansen KR, Peck JD, Coward RM, Wild RA, Trussell JC, Krawetz SA, et al. Intrauterine insemination performance characteristics and post-processing total motile sperm count in relation to live birth for couples with unexplained infertility in a randomised, multicentre clinical trial. Hum Reprod. 2020;35(6):1296-305.

29. Immediata V, Patrizio P, Parisen Toldin MR, Morenghi E, Ronchetti C, Cirillo F, et al. Twenty-one year experience with intrauterine inseminations after controlled ovarian stimulation with gonadotropins: maternal age is the only prognostic factor for success. J Assist Reprod Genet. 2020;37(5):1195-201.

30. Pellicer A, Simon C, Remoh J. Effects of aging on the female reproductive system. Hum Reprod. 1995;10 Suppl 2:77-83.

31. Cano F, Simon C, Remoh J, Pellicer A. Effect of aging on the female reproductive system: evidence for a role of uterine senescence in the decline in female fecundity. Fertil

Steril. 1995;64(3):584-9.

32. Shirasuna K, Iwata H. Effect of aging on the female reproductive function. Contracept Reprod Med. 2017;2:23.

33. Ferraretti AP, Nygren K, Andersen AN, De Mouzon J, Kupka M, Calhaz Jorge C, et al. Trends over 15 years in ART in europe: an analysis of 6 million cyclest. Hum Reprod Open. 2017;2017(2):12.

34. Badawy A, Elnashar A, Eltotongy M. Effect of sperm morphology and number on success of intrauterine insemination. Fertil Steril. 2009;91(3):777-81.

35. Kamath MS, Bhave P, Aleyamma T, Nair R, Chandy A, Mangalaraj AM, et al. Predictive factors for pregnancy after intrauterine insemination: a prospective study of factors affecting outcome. J Hum Reprod Sci. 2010;3(3):129-34.

36. Nuojua Huttunen S, Tomas C, Bloigu R, Tuomivaara L, Martikainen H. Intrauterine insemination treatment in subfertility: an analysis of factors affecting outcome. Hum Reprod. 1999;14(3):698-703.

37. Plosker SM, Jacobson W, Amato P. Predicting and optimizing success in an intrauterine insemination programme. Hum Reprod. 1994;9(11):2014-21.

38. Frederick JL, Denker MS, Rojas A, Horta I, Stone SC, Asch RH, et al. Is there a role for ovarian stimulation and intra-uterine insemination after age 40? Hum Reprod. 1994;9(12):2284-6.

39. Sahakyan M, Harlow BL, Hornstein MD. Influence of age, diagnosis, and cycle number on pregnancy rates with gonadotropin-induced controlled ovarian hyperstimulation and intrauterine insemination. Fertil Steril. 1999;72(3):500-4.

40. Dickey RP, Pyrzak R, Lu PY, Taylor SN, Rye PH. Comparison of the sperm quality necessary for successful intrauterine insemination with world health organization threshold values for normal sperm. Fertil Steril. 1999;71(4):684-9.

41. Houmard BS, Juang MP, Soules MR, Fujimoto VY. Factors influencing pregnancy rates with a combined clomiphene citrate/gonadotropin protocol for nonassisted reproductive technology fertility treatment. Fertil Steril. 2002;77(2):384-6.

42. Belloc S, Cohen Bacrie P, Benkhalifa M, Cohen Bacrie M, De Mouzon J, Hazout A, et al. Effect of maternal and paternal age on pregnancy and miscarriage rates after intrauterine insemination. Reprod Biomed Online. 2008;17(3):392-7.

43. Stone BA, Vargyas JM, Ringler GE, Stein AL, Marrs RP. Determinants of the outcome of intrauterine insemination: analysis of outcomes of 9963 consecutive cycles. Am J Obstet Gynecol. 1999;180(6):1522-34.

44. Vargas Tominaga L, Alarcon F, Vargas A, Bernal G, Medina A, Polo Z. Associated factors to pregnancy in intrauterine insemination. JBRA Assist Reprod. 2020;24(1):66-9.

45. Abdalla HI, Burton G, Kirkland A, Johnson MR, Leonard T, Brooks AA, et al. Age, pregnancy and miscarriage: uterine versus ovarian factors. Hum Reprod. 1993;8(9):1512-7.

46. Khalil MR, Rasmussen PE, Erb K, Laursen SB, Rex S, Westergaard LG. Homologous intrauterine insemination. An evaluation of prognostic factors based on a review of 2473 cycles. Acta Obstet Gynecol Scand. 2001;80(1):74-81.

47. Mathieu C, Ecochard R, Bied V, Lornage J, Czyba JC. Cumulative conception rate following intrauterine artificial insemination with husband's spermatozoa: influence of husband's age. Hum Reprod. 1995;10(5):1090-7.

48. Iberico G, Vioque J, Ariza N, Lozano JM, Roca M, Llacer J, et al. Analysis of factors influencing pregnancy rates in homologous intrauterine insemination. Fertil Steril. 2004;81(5):1308-13.

49. Ahinko Hakamaa K, Huhtala H, Tinkanen H. Success in intrauterine insemination: the role of etiology. Acta Obstet Gynecol Scand. 2007;86(7):855-60.

50. Erdem A, Erdem M, Atmaca S, Korucuoglu U, Karabacak O. Factors affecting live birth rate in intrauterine insemination cycles with recombinant gonadotropin stimulation. Reprod Biomed Online. 2008;17(2):199-206.

51. Erdem M, Erdem A, Mutlu MF, Ozisik S, Yildiz S, Guler I, et al. The impact of sperm morphology on the outcome of intrauterine insemination cycles with gonadotropins in unexplained and male subfertility. Eur J Obstet Gynecol Reprod Biol. 2016;197:120-4.

52. Buyalos RP, Daneshmand S, Brzechffa PR. Basal estradiol and folliclestimulating hormone predict fecundity in women of advanced reproductive age undergoing ovulation induction therapy. Fertil Steril. 1997;68(2):272-7.

53. Navot D, Bergh PA, Williams MA, Garrisi GJ, Guzman I, Sandler B, et al. Poor oocyte quality rather than implantation failure as a cause of age-related decline in female fertility. Lancet. 1991;337(8754):1375-7.

54. Ahmed Ebbiary NA, Lenton EA, Salt C, Ward AM, Cooke ID. The significance of elevated basal follicle stimulating hormone in regularly menstruating infertile women. Hum Reprod. 1994;9(2):245-52.

55. Mullin CM, Trivax B, Baxter M, Virji N, Saketos M, San Roman G. Day 3 follicle stimulating hormone (FSH) and estradiol (E2): could these values be used as markers to predict pregnancy outcomes in women undergoing ovulation induction (OI) therapy with intrauterine insemination (IUI) cycles? Fertil Steril. 2005;84:162.

56. Soria M, Pradillo G, Garda J, Ramon P, Castillo A, Jordana C, et al. Pregnancy predictors after intrauterine insemination: analysis of 3012 cycles in 1201 couples. J Reprod Infertil. 2012;13(3):158-66.

57. Boulard V, Charbit B, Brasseur F, Lourdel E, Copin H, Merviel P. Prognostic factors of pregnancy in intrauterine insemination with sperm of donor: a review of 535 cycles over 7 years. J Gynecol Obstet Biol Reprod. 2013;42(1):40-8.

58. Yavuz A, Demirci O, Sozen H, Uludogan M. Predictive factors influencing pregnancy rates after intrauterine insemination. Iran J Reprod Med. 2013;11(3):227 -34.

59. Bakas P, Boutas I, Creatsa M, Vlahos N, Gregoriou O, Creatsas G, et al. Can anti-mullerian hormone (AMH) predict the outcome of intrauterine insemination with controlled ovarian stimulation? Gynecol Endocrinol. 2015;31(10):765-8.

60. Moro F, Tropea A, Scarinci E, Leoncini E, Boccia S, Federico A, et al. Anti- mullerian hormone concentrations and antral follicle counts for the prediction of pregnancy outcomes after intrauterine insemination. Int J Gynaecol Obstet. 2016;133(1):64-8.

61. Lamazou F, Fuchs F, Genro V, Malagrida L, Torre A, Albert M, et al. Predictive value of antimullerian hormone on outcomes of intrauterine inseminations. J Gynecol Obstet Biol Reprod. 2012;41(2):122-7.

62. Dondik Y, Virji N, Butler TS, Gaskins JT, Pagidas K, Sung L. The value of anti- mullerian hormone in predicting clinical pregnancy after intrauterine insemination. J Obstet Gynaecol Can. 2017;39(10):880-5.

63. Broer SL, Broekmans FM, Laven JE, Fauser BM. Anti-mullerian hormone: ovarian reserve testing and its potential clinical implications. Hum Reprod Update. 2014;20(5):688-701.

64. Dosso N, Robin G, Catteau Jonard S, Pigny P, Leroy Billiard M, Dewailly D. Impact of plasma anti-mullerian hormone levels on the results of assisted reproduction techniques. Single-centre retrospective analysis of 2011 cycles (ICSI indications and bilateral tubal obstructions excluded). J Gynecol Obstet Biol Reprod. 2015;44(1):63-71.

65. Moreau J, Gatimel N, Simon C, Cohade C, Lesourd F, Parinaud J, et al. Agespecific anti-mullerian hormone (AMH) levels poorly affects cumulative live birth rate after intrauterine insemination. Eur J Obstet Gynecol Reprod Biol X. 2019;3:100043.

66. Tremellen K, Kolo M. Serum anti-mullerian hormone is a useful measure of quantitative ovarian reserve but does not predict the chances of live-birth pregnancy. Aust N Z J Obstet Gynaecol. 2010;50(6):568-72.

67. Hendin BN, Falcone T, Hallak J, Nelson DR, Vemullapalli S, Goldberg J, et al. The effect of patient and semen characteristics on live birth rates following intrauterine insemination: a retrospective study. J Assist Reprod Genet. 2000;17(5):245-52.

68. Montanaro Gauci M, Kruger TF, Coetzee K, Smith K, Van Der Merwe JP, Lombard CJ. Stepwise regression analysis to study male and female factors impacting on pregnancy rate in an intrauterine insemination programme. Andrologia. 2001;33(3):135-41.

69. Lee VS, Wong JY, Loh SE, Leong NY. Sperm motility in the semen analysis affects the outcome of superovulation intrauterine insemination in the treatment of infertile asian couples with male factor infertility. Int J Gynaecol Obstet. 2002;109(2):115-20.

70. Zhao Y, Vlahos N, Wyncott D, Petrella C, Garcia J, Zacur H, et al. Impact of semen characteristics on the success of intrauterine insemination. J Assist Reprod Genet. 2004;21(5):143-8.

71. Yalti S, Gurbuz B, Sezer H, Celik S. Effects of semen characteristics on IUI combined with mild ovarian stimulation. Arch Androl. 2004;50(4):239-46.

72. Haim D, Leniaud L, Porcher R, Martin Pont B, Wolf JP, Sifer C. Prospective evaluation of the impact of sperm characteristics on the outcome of intrauterine insemination. Gynecol Obstet Fertil. 2009;37(3):229-35.

73. Jellad S, Basly M, Chibani M, Rachdi R. Predictive factors for intrauterine insemination success: analysis of semen parameters affecting outcome. Internet J Urol. 2014;12:1-7.

74. Kdous M, Kacem K, Ellouze S, Elloumi H, Khrouf M, Chaker A, et al. Threshold levels of sperm parameters impacting on pregnancy rate in an intrauterine insemination programme. Donn J Med Lab Diagn. 2015;1:19-23.

75. Mollaahmadi L, Keramat A, Ghiasi A, Hashemzadeh M. The relationship between semen parameters in processed and unprocessed semen with intrauterine insemination success rates. J Turk Ger Gynecol Assoc. 2019;20(1):1-7.

76. Ainsworth AJ, Barnard EP, Baumgarten SC, Weaver AL, Khan Z. Intrauterine insemination cycles: prediction of success and thresholds for poor prognosis and futile care. J Assist Reprod Genet. 2020;37(10):2435-42.

77. Mankus EB, Holden AE, Seeker PM, Kampschmidt JC, McLaughlin JE, Schenken RS, et al. Prewash total motile count is a poor predictor of live birth in intrauterine insemination cycles. Fertil Steril. 2019;111(4):708-13.

78. Wainer R, Albert M, Dorion A, Bailly M, Bergere M, Lombroso R, et al. Influence of the number of motile spermatozoa inseminated and of their morphology on the success of intrauterine insemination. Hum Reprod. 2004;19(9):2060-5.

79. Miller DC, Hollenbeck BK, Smith GD, Randolph JF, Christman GM, Smith YR, et al. Processed total motile sperm count correlates with pregnancy outcome after intrauterine insemination. Urology. 2002;60(3):497-501.

80. Van Weert JM, Repping S, Van Voorhis BJ, Van Der Veen F, Bossuyt PM, Mol BJ. Performance of the postwash total motile sperm count as a predictor of pregnancy at the time of intrauterine insemination: a meta-analysis. Fertil Steril. 2004;82(3):612 -20.

81. Gubert PG, Pudwell J, Van Vugt D, Reid RL, Velez MP. Number of motile spermatozoa

inseminated and pregnancy outcomes in intrauterine insemination. Fertil Res Pract. 2019;5:10.

82. Demir B, Dilbaz B, Cinar O, Karadag B, Tasci Y, Kocak M, et al. Factors affecting pregnancy outcome of intrauterine insemination cycles in couples with favourable female characteristics. J Obstet Gynaecol. 2011;31(5):420-3.

83. Muthigi A, Jahandideh S, Bishop LA, Naeemi FK, Shipley SK, O'brien JE, et al. Clarifying the relationship between total motile sperm counts and intrauterine insemination pregnancy rates. Fertil Steril. 2021;115(6):1454-60.

84. Starosta A, Gordon CE, Hornstein MD. Predictive factors for intrauterine insemination outcomes: a review. Fertil Res Pract. 2020;6(1):23.

85. Hassan N, Agbo C, Dahan MH. Pregnancy rates unaffected by sperm count in intrauterine insemination: a retrospective cohort study. Minerva Ginecol. 2017;69(1):6-12.

86. Delaroche L, Caillou H, Lamazou F, Genauzeau E, Meicler P, Oger P, et al. Live birth after intrauterine insemination: is there an upper cut-off for the number of motile spermatozoa inseminated? Reprod Biomed Online. 2021;42(1):117-24.

87. Ombelet W, Vandeput H, Van De Putte G, Cox A, Janssen M, Jacobs P, et al. Intrauterine insemination after ovarian stimulation with clomiphene citrate: predictive potential of inseminating motile count and sperm morphology. Hum Reprod. 1997;12(7):1458-63.

88. Cohlen BJ, Velde ER, Van Kooij RJ, Looman CW, Habbema JD. Controlled ovarian hyperstimulation and intrauterine insemination for treating male subfertility: a controlled study. Hum Reprod. 1998;13(6):1553-3.

89. Tomlinson M, Lewis S, Morroll D. Sperm quality and its relationship to natural and assisted conception: british fertility society guidelines for practice. Hum Fertil. 2013;16(3):175-93.

90. Hauser R, Yogev L, Botchan A, Lessing JB, Paz G, Yavetz H. Intrauterine insemination in male factor subfertility: significance of sperm motility and morphology assessed by strict criteria. Andrologia. 2001;33(1):13-7.

91. Van Waart J, Kruger TF, Lombard CJ, Ombelet W. Predictive value of normal sperm morphology in intrauterine nsemination (IUI): a structured literature review. Hum Reprod Update. 2001;7(5):495-500.

92. Shibahara H, Obara H, Ayustawati, Hirano Y, Suzuki T, Ohno A, et al. Prediction of pregnancy by intrauterine insemination using CASA estimates and strict criteria in patients with male factor infertility. Int J Androl. 2004;27(2):63-8.

93. Nikbakht R, Saharkhiz N. The influence of sperm morphology, total motile sperm count of semen and the number of motile sperm inseminated in sperm samples on the success of intrauterine insemination. Int J Fertil Steril. 2011;5(3):168-73.

94. Karabinus DS, Gelety TJ. The impact of sperm morphology evaluated by strict criteria on intrauterine insemination success. Fertil Steril. 1997;67(3):536-41.

95. Sun Y, Li B, Fan LQ, Zhu WB, Chen XJ, Feng JH, et al. Does sperm morphology affect the outcome of intrauterine insemination in patients with normal sperm concentration and motility? Andrologia. 2012;44(5):299-304.

96. Deveneau NE, Sinno O, Krause M, Eastwood D, Sandlow JI, Robb P, et al. Impact of sperm morphology on the likelihood of pregnancy after intrauterine insemination. Fertil Steril. 2014;102(6):1584-90.

97. Kohn TP, Kohn JR, Ramasamy R. Effect of sperm morphology on pregnancy success via intrauterine insemination: a systematic review and meta-analysis. J Urol. 2018;199(3):812-

22.

98. Zinaman MJ, Brown CC, Selevan SG, Clegg ED. Semen quality and human fertility: a prospective study with healthy couples. J Androl. 2000;21(1):145-53.

99. Kunzle R, Mueller MD, Hanggi W, Birkhauser MH, Drescher H, Bersinger NA. Semen quality of male smokers and nonsmokers in infertile couples. Fertil Steril. 2003;79(2):287-91.

100. Lewin A, Gonen O, Orvieto R, Schenker JG. Effect of smoking on concentration, motility and zona-free hamster test on human sperm. Arch Androl. 1991;27(1):51-4.

101. Adelusi B, Al Twaijiri MH, Al Meshari A, Kangave D, Al Nuaim LA, Younnus B. Correlation of smoking and coffee drinking with sperm progressive motility in infertile males. Afr J Med Med Sci. 1998;27(1-2):47-50.

102. Brugo Olmedo S, Chillik C, Kopelman S. Definition and causes of infertility. Reprod Biomed Online. 2001;2(1):41-53.

103. Practice Committee of American Society for Reproductive Medicine. Smoking and infertility. Fertil Steril. 2008;90 Suppl 5:254-9.

104. Tomlinson MJ, Amissah Arthur JB, Thompson KA, Kasraie JL, Bentick B. Prognostic indicators for intrauterine insemination (IUI): statistical model for IUI success. Hum Reprod. 1996;11(9):1892-6.

105. Steures P, Van Der Steeg JW, Verhoeve HR, Van Dop PA, Hompes PA, Bossuyt PM, et al. Does ovarian hyperstimulation in intrauterine insemination for cervical factor subfertility improve pregnancy rates? Hum Reprod. 2004;19(10):2263-6.

106. Ashrafi M, Rashidi M, Ghasemi A, Arabipoor A, Daghighi S, Pourasghari P, et al. The role of infertility etiology in success rate of intrauterine insemination cycles: an evaluation of predictive factors for pregnancy rate. Int J Fertil Steril. 2013;7(2):100-7.

107. Cao S, Zhao C, Zhang J, Wu X, Zhou L, Guo X, et al. A minimum number of motile spermatozoa are required for successful fertilization through artificial intrauterine insemination with husband's spermatozoa. Andrologia. 2014;46(5):529- 34.

108. Ghaffari F, Sadatmahalleh SJ, Akhoond MR, Eftekhari Yazdi P, Zolfaghari Z. Evaluating the effective factors in pregnancy after intrauterine insemination: a retrospective study. Int J Fertil Steril. 2015;9(3):300-8.

109. Kerin JF, Kirby C, Peek J, Jeffrey R, Warnes GM, Matthews CD, et al. Improved conception rate after intrauterine insemination of washed spermatozoa from men with poor semen quality. Lancet. 1984;1(8376):533-5.

110. Cabry Goubet R, Scheffler F, Belhadri Mansouri N, Belloc S, Lourdel E, Devaux A, et al. Effect of gonadotropin types and indications on homologous intrauterine insemination success: a study from 1251 cycles and a review of the literature. Biomed Res Int. 2017;2017:3512784.

111. Haller L, Severac F, Rongieres C, Ohl J, Bettahar K, Lichtblau I, et al. Intrauterine insemination 24 or 48 hours after ovulation: pregnancy and delivery rates. Gynecol Obstet Fertil Senol. 2017;45(4):210-4.

112. Sicchieri F, Silva AB, Silva AJ, Navarro PA, Ferriani RA, Reis RD. Prognostic factors in intrauterine insemination cycles. JBRA Assist Reprod. 2018;22(1):2-7.

113. Rotterdam ESHRE/ASRM-Sponsored PCOS Consensus Workshop Group. Revised 2003 consensus on diagnostic criteria and long-term health risks related to polycystic ovary syndrome. Fertil Steril. 2004;81(1):19-25.

114. Thessaloniki ESHRE/ASRM-Sponsored PCOS Consensus Workshop Group. Consensus on infertility treatment related to polycystic ovary syndrome. Hum Reprod. 2008;23(3):462-77.

115.   Merviel P, Bouee S, Menard M, Le Martelot MT, Roche S, Lelievre C, et al. Which ovarian stimulation to which women: the polycystic ovary syndrome (PCOS). Gynecol Obstet Fertil Senol. 2017;45(11):623-31.

116.   Evers JH. Female subfertility. Lancet. 2002;360(9327):151-9.

117.   O'flynn N. Assessment and treatment for people with fertility problems: NICE guideline. Br J Gen Pract. 2014;64(618):50-1.

118.   Nandi A, Gudi A, Shah A, Homburg R. An online survey of specialists' opinion on first line management options for unexplained subfertility. Hum Fertil. 2015;18(1):48-53.

119.   Farquhar CM, Liu E, Armstrong S, Arroll N, Lensen S, Brown J. Intrauterine insemination with ovarian stimulation versus expectant management for unexplained infertility (TUI): a pragmatic, open-label, randomised, controlled, two-centre trial. Lancet. 2018;391(10119):441-50.

120.   Bensdorp AJ, Cohlen BJ, Heineman MJ, Vandekerckhove P. Intra-uterine insemination for male subfertility. Cochrane Database Syst Rev. 2007 Oct 17;(4):CD000360.

121.   Bensdorp AJ, Tjon Kon Fat RI, Bossuyt PM, Koks CM, Oosterhuis GE, Hoek A, et al. Prevention of multiple pregnancies in couples with unexplained or mild male subfertility: randomised controlled trial of in vitro fertilisation with single embryo transfer or in vitro fertilisation in modified natural cycle compared with intrauterine insemination with controlled ovarian hyperstimulation. Br Med J. 2015;350:g7771.

122.   Cochet T, Gatimel N, Moreau J, Cohade C, Fajau C, Lesourd F, et al. Effect of unilateral tubal abnormalities on the results of intrauterine inseminations. Reprod Biomed Online. 2017;35(3):314-7.

123.   Berker B, Kahraman K, Taskin S, Sukur YE, Sonmezer M, Atabekoglu CS. Recombinant FSH versus clomiphene citrate for ovarian stimulation in couples with unexplained infertility and male subfertility undergoing intrauterine insemination: a randomized trial. Arch Gynecol Obstet. 2011;284(6):1561-6.

124.   Lin MH, Hwu YM, Lin SY, Lee RK. Treatment of infertile women with unilateral tubal occlusion by intrauterine insemination and ovarian stimulation. Taiwan J Obstet Gynecol. 2013;52(3):360-4.

125.   Yi G, Jee BC, Suh CS, Kim SH. Stimulated intrauterine insemination in women with unilateral tubal occlusion. Clin Exp Reprod Med. 2012;39(2):68-72.

126.   Collinet P, Fritel X, Revel Delhom C, Ballester M, Bolze PA, Borghese B, et al. Management of endometriosis: CNGCF/HAS clinical practice guidelines - short version. J Gynecol Obstet Hum Reprod. 2018;47(7):265-74.

127.   Cosma S, Benedetto C. Classification algorithm of patients with endometriosis: Proposal for tailored management. Adv Clin Exp Med. 2020;29(5):615-22.

128.   Van Der Houwen LE, Schreurs AF, Schats R, Heymans MW, Lambalk CB, Hompes PA, et al. Efficacy and safety of intrauterine insemination in patients with moderate-to-severe endometriosis. Reprod Biomed Online. 2014;28(5):590-8.

129.   Biljan MM, Mahutte NG, Tulandi T, Tan SL. Prospective randomized doubleblind trial of the correlation between time of administration and antiestrogenic effects of clomiphene citrate on reproductive end organs. Fertil Steril. 1999;71(4):633-8.

130.   Cantineau AP, Cohlen BJ, Heineman MJ. Ovarian stimulation protocols (antioestrogens, gonadotrophins with and without GnRH agonists/antagonists) for intrauterine insemination (IUI) in women with subfertility. Cochrane Database Syst Rev. 2007 Apr 18;(2):CD005356.

131.   Arici A, Byrd W, Bradshaw K, Kutteh WH, Marshburn P, Carr BR. Evaluation of

clomiphene citrate and human chorionic gonadotropin treatment: a prospective, randomized, crossover study during intrauterine insemination cycles. Fertil Steril. 1994;61(2):314-8.

132.	Martinez AR, Bernardus RE, Voorhorst FJ, Vermeiden JP, Schoemaker J. Intrauterine insemination does and clomiphene citrate does not improve fecundity in couples with infertility due to male or idiopathic factors: a prospective, randomized, controlled study. Fertil Steril. 1990;53(5):847-53.

133.	Weiss NS, Van Vliet MN, Limpens J, Hompes PA, Lambalk CB, Mochtar MH, et al. Endometrial thickness in women undergoing IUI with ovarian stimulation. How thick is too thin? A systematic review and meta-analysis. Hum Reprod. 2017;32(5):1009-18.

134.	Danhof NA, Van Wely M, Repping S, Koks C, Verhoeve HR, De Bruin JP, et al. Follicle stimulating hormone versus clomiphene citrate in intrauterine insemination for unexplained subfertility: a randomized controlled trial. Hum Reprod. 2018;33(10):1866-74.

135.	Mitwally MF, Casper RF. Use of an aromatase inhibitor for induction of ovulation in patients with an inadequate response to clomiphene citrate. Fertil Steril. 2001;75(2):305-9.

136.	Badawy A, Elnashar A, Totongy M. Clomiphene citrate or aromatase inhibitors combined with gonadotropins for superovulation in women undergoing intrauterine insemination: a prospective randomised trial. J Obstet Gynaecol. 2010;30(6):617-21.

137.	Huang S, Du X, Wang R, Li R, Wang H, Luo L, et al. Ovulation induction and intrauterine insemination in infertile women with polycystic ovary syndrome: a comparison of drugs. Eur J Obstet Gynecol Reprod Biol. 2018;231:117-21.

138.	Nguyen TT, Doan HT, Quan LH, Lam NM. Effect of letrozole for ovulation induction combined with intrauterine insemination on women with polycystic ovary syndrome. Gynecol Endocrinol. 2020;36(10):860-3.

139.	Legro RS, Brzyski RG, Diamond MP, Coutifaris C, Schlaff WD, Casson P, et al. Letrozole versus clomiphene for infertility in the polycystic ovary syndrome. N Engl J Med. 2014;371(2):119-29.

140.	Franik S, Eltrop SM, Kremer JA, Kiesel L, Farquhar C. Aromatase inhibitors (letrozole) for subfertile women with polycystic ovary syndrome. Cochrane Database Syst Rev. 2018 May 24;5(5):CD010287.

141.	Yun BH, Chon SJ, Park JH, Seo SK, Cho S, Choi YS, et al. Minimal stimulation using gonadotropin combined with clomiphene citrate or letrozole for intrauterine insemination. Yonsei Med J. 2015;56(2):490-6.

142.	Van Rumste ME, Custers IM, Van Der Veen F, Van Wely M, Evers JH, Mol BJ. The influence of the number of follicles on pregnancy rates in intrauterine insemination with ovarian stimulation: a meta-analysis. Hum Reprod Update. 2008;14(6):563-70.

143.	Esmailzadeh S, Faramarzi M. Endometrial thickness and pregnancy outcome after intrauterine insemination. Fertil Steril. 2007;88(2):432-7.

144.	Danhof NA, Van Eekelen R, Repping S, Mol BJ, Van Der Veen F, Van Wely M, et al. Endometrial thickness as a biomarker for ongoing pregnancy in IUI for unexplained subfertility: a secondary analysis. Hum Reprod Open. 2020;2020(1):24.

145.	Cohlen B, Bijkerk A, Van Der Poel S, Ombelet W. IUI: review and systematic assessment of the evidence that supports global recommendations. Hum Reprod Update. 2018;24(3):300-19.

146.	Claman P, Wilkie V, Collins D. Timing intrauterine insemination either 33 or 39 hours after administration of human chorionic gonadotropin yields the same pregnancy rates as after superovulation therapy. Fertil Steril. 2004;82(1):13-6.

147.	Rahman SM, Karmakar D, Malhotra N, Kumar S. Timing of intrauterine insemination:

an attempt to unravel the enigma. Arch Gynecol Obstet. 2011;284(4):1023-7.

148. Aydin Y, Hassa H, Oge T, Tokgoz VY. A randomized study of simultaneous hCG administration with intrauterine insemination in stimulated cycles. Eur J Obstet Gynecol Reprod Biol. 2013;170(2):444-8.

149. Lee J, Hwang S, Lee J, Yoo J, Jang D, Hwang K, et al. Effect of insemination timing on pregnancy outcome in association with female age, sperm motility, sperm morphology and sperm concentration in intrauterine insemination. J Obstet Gynaecol Res. 2018;44(6):1100-6.

150. Ragni G, Maggioni P, Guermandi E, Testa A, Baroni E, Colombo M, et al. Efficacy of double intrauterine insemination in controlled ovarian hyperstimulation cycles. Fertil Steril. 1999;72(4):619-22.

151. Osuna C, Matorras R, Pijoan JI, Rodnguez Escudero FJ. One versus two inseminations per cycle in intrauterine insemination with sperm from patients' husbands: a systematic review of the literature. Fertil Steril. 2004;82(1):17-24.

152. Marshburn PB, Giddings A, Causby S, Matthews ML, Usadi RS, Steuerwald N, et al. Influence of ejaculatory abstinence on seminal total antioxidant capacity and sperm membrane lipid peroxidation. Fertil Steril. 2014;102(3):705-10.

153. Bahadur G, Homburg R, Muneer A, Racich P, Alangaden T, Al Habib A, et al. First line fertility treatment strategies regarding IUI and IVF require clinical evidence. Hum Reprod. 2016;31(6):1141-6.

154. Jurema MW, Vieira AD, Bankowski B, Petrella C, Zhao Y, Wallach E, et al. Effect of ejaculatory abstinence period on the pregnancy rate after intrauterine insemination. Fertil Steril. 2005;84(3):678-81.

155. Practice Committee of the American Society for Reproductive Medicine. Performing the embryo transfer: a guideline. Fertil Steril. 2017;107(4):882-96.

156. Van Der Poel N, Farquhar C, Abou Setta AM, Benschop L, Heineman MJ. Soft versus firm catheters for intrauterine insemination. Cochrane Database Syst Rev. 2010 Nov 10;(11):CD006225.

157. Khan SN, Storer BL, Peck JD, Goddard LD, Hansen KR, Craig LB. Does a difficult intrauterine insemination ower pregnancy rates and live birth rates? Fertil Steril. 2013;100(3):378.

158. Hubayter ZR, Muasher SJ. Luteal supplementation in in vitro fertilization: more questions than answers. Fertil Steril. 2008;89(4):749-58.

159. Van Der Linden M, Buckingham K, Farquhar C, Kremer JM, Metwally M. Luteal phase support for assisted reproduction cycles. Cochrane Database Syst Rev. 2015 Jul 7;2015(7):CD009154.

160. Green KA, Zolton JR, Schermerhorn SV, Lewis TD, Healy MW, Terry N, et al. Progesterone luteal support after ovulation induction and intrauterine insemination: an updated systematic review and meta-analysis. Fertil Steril. 2017;107(4):924-33.

161. Dupuis S, Dani V, Fatfouta I, Staccini P, Delotte J. Impact du soutien de la phase luteale par human chorionic gonadotropine (hCG) dans les inseminations intra- uterines. Gynecol Obstet Fertil Senol. 2019;47(10):739-46.

162. Scher AI, Petterson B, Blair E, Ellenberg JH, Grether JK, Haan E, et al. The risk of mortality or cerebral palsy in twins: a collaborative population-based study. Pediatr Res. 2002;52(5):671-81.

163. Santana DS, Cecatti JG, Surita FG, Silveira C, Costa ML, Souza JP, et al. Twin pregnancy and severe maternal outcomes: the world health organization multicountry survey

on maternal and newborn health. Obstet Gynecol. 2016;127(4):631-41.

164.	Ombelet W, De Sutter P, Van Der Elst J, Martens G. Multiple gestation and infertility treatment: registration, reflection and reaction--the belgian project. Hum Reprod Update. 2005;11(1):3-14.

165.	Aboulghar M, Mansour R, Serour G, Abdrazek A, Amin Y, Rhodes C. Controlled ovarian hyperstimulation and intrauterine insemination for treatment of unexplained infertility should be limited to a maximum of three trials. Fertil Steril. 2001;75(1):88- 91.

65

Resume

Introduction :

Intrauterine insemination (IUI) is the simplest and least expensive method of medically assisted procreation (MAP), often used as a first-line treatment, particularly in cases of unexplained hypofertility. However, its results remain disappointing.

The aim of this study was to determine the factors predicting the success of IUI cycles in order to better select candidates for this MPA technique.

Methods :

This was a retrospective study conducted at the reproductive health service of the main military training hospital in Tunis over a 4-year period, between January 2016 and January 2020. We included in this study 196 infertile couples receiving IUI cycles during this period whose age was <40 years with at least one tube permeable to hysterosalpingography and a final progressive motile sperm count >1 million. The criterion for judgement was the clinical pregnancy rate.

Results:

Three hundred and twenty-eight IUI attempts were analysed. The overall clinical pregnancy rate was 15.2%. The maximum number of pregnancies was observed in women with polycystic ovary syndrome (35.1%). The duration of infertility had a significant impact on the pregnancy rate. Prolonging the duration of infertility beyond 6 years was a negative predictor of pregnancy after IUI (p=0.02). A basal FSH level of less than 7 IU/ml was associated with a successful IUI attempt (p=0.016). Initial total and progressive mobility >40% on the day of insemination were associated with a significant increase in pregnancy rates (p=0.002 and p=0.001 respectively). The chances of a successful IUI cycle were greater when the total number of progressive motile sperm inseminated exceeded 5 million (17.9% versus 5.3%, p=0.007). A significant increase in the pregnancy rate was noted when the percentage of typical forms exceeded 15% (p=0.001). Moving from 1 to 2 or more follicles increased the chance of pregnancy from 8.6% to 18.8% (**p=0**.015). Similarly, the pregnancy rate was significantly higher when the thickness of the endometrium was greater than or equal to 9mm (38.8% vs 15.2%, p=0.001).

Conclusion:

Our results suggest that certain male and female factors influence the outcome of attempts. Taking these parameters into account will enable us to provide couples with better guidance, and thus optimise their chances of IUI success.

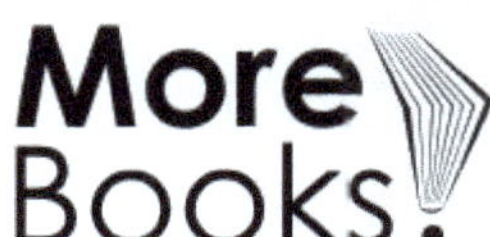

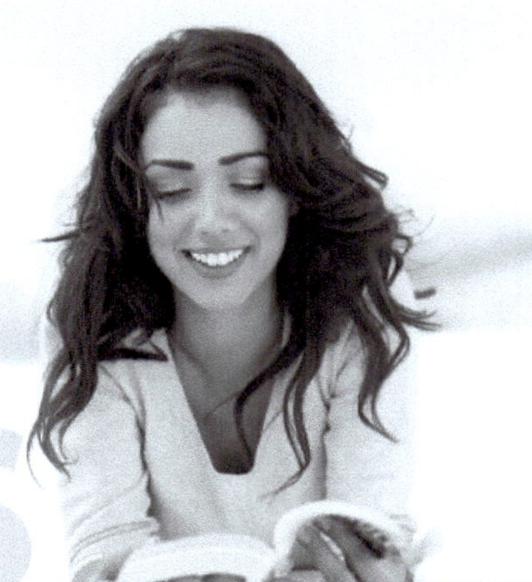

yes
I want morebooks!

Buy your books fast and straightforward online - at one of world's fastest growing online book stores! Environmentally sound due to Print-on-Demand technologies.

Buy your books online at
www.morebooks.shop

Kaufen Sie Ihre Bücher schnell und unkompliziert online – auf einer der am schnellsten wachsenden Buchhandelsplattformen weltweit! Dank Print-On-Demand umwelt- und ressourcenschonend produziert.

Bücher schneller online kaufen
www.morebooks.shop

info@omniscriptum.com
www.omniscriptum.com

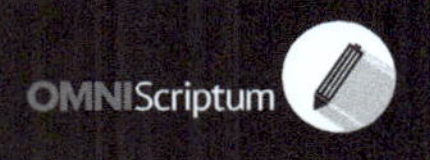

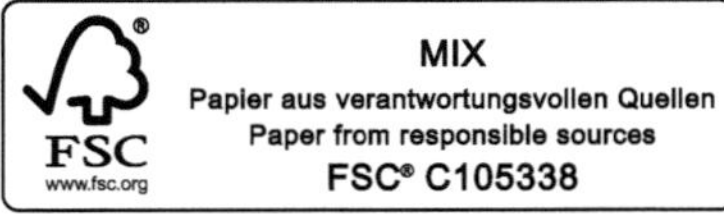

Printed by Books on Demand GmbH, Norderstedt / Germany